THE NO DIET-DIET

First published by Howarth Press,
Suite 16 Brooklands House, Marlborough House,
Lancing, West Sussex, BN15 8AF.

ISBN-13 978-1456524579

ISBN-10 1456524577

This book gives non-specific, general advice and should not be relied on as a substitute for proper medical conslutation. The author and publisher cannot accept responsibility for illness arising out of the failure to seek medical advice from a doctor. or healthcare professional.

CONTENTS

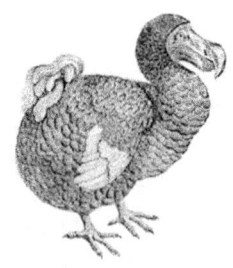

"Come to the edge."
"We might fall."
"Come to the edge."
"It's too high..."
"COME TO THE EDGE!"
So they came
And he pushed
And they flew.

Christopher Logue, From Ode to the Dodo.
Turret Books, 36 Great Queen Street, London WC2B 5A

ACKNOWLEDGEMENTS

This book was made possible by the loving support and encouragement of the following people:

My wife Jane and children Lucy-Jane and James whose love is manifested in many ways, especially in their encouragement, patience and understanding.
For a young family the most precious commodity they have is their time together, and they gave willingly more of that time than I deserve, or indeed hoped for to pursue this work.

My colleagues, Angela & John, Anna & Martin, Suzi, Jeremy and Alan who have contributed so much, offered support, help advice and encouragement throughout the long and sometimes challenging development of this programme.

And finally to my parents Jim and Lil and brother David who have been role models of the highest quality.

Thank you all.

Eat what you desire and still lose weight

If you would like to eat what you want, be free of counting calories or just eat and drink the things you enjoy - and still lose weight - you will find out how to do so by using the techniques in this programme.

The No Diet-Diet is not a traditional weight loss programme. There are no restricted foods, you are free to eat exactly what you want.

If you have tried, and failed to lose weight in the past this can actually be an advantage. Your previous attempts to lose weight have not been wasted. This is because the experience that you have gained will have given you a valuable insight into why and how you can sucessfully lose weight now. In one of the few comprehensive studies conducted on weight loss, it was found that people who had been unsuccessful in losing weight in the past were 15% more likely succeed in the future.

Your previous failure has taught you many valuable lessions. For example; you already know exactly which foods to eat, and which to avoid. You also know exactly how much you should eat to lose weight. Your body already tells you which foods make you feel healthy by making you feel good about yourself - as well as telling you which foods are bad for you by leaving you feeling guilty or bloated after eating them.

This inner knowledge, was observed in a remarkable experiment, where a group of children were given the opportunity to eat anything they wanted. For three weeks they had absolute control over their diet, at first all they ate was complete junk, sweets, snacks and fast foods. But during the course of the three week experiment a remarkable change was observed. The children switched to eating healthy foods. Salads and fish steadily replaced the chips and burgers. Ordinary water became more popular than cola. Sweets, crisps and snacks were not being touched.

The conclusion drawn from this experiment was that the children instinctively knew which foods were good for them in the long term. It is only outside pressures that confuse this knowledge. Exactly the same is true for you and me.

With the knowledge that you already possess, and by following the simple techniques outlined in this book, you can start on the process of losing weight - without having consciously to restrict the amount or type of food you eat.

You can easily tap into this wealth of knowledge right now. The technique used to do this is called visualisation - which is just a way to unlock the accumulated information already stored inside your head.

Visualisation requires no special skill or discipline, although like every skill you have mastered, the more you practice it the easier it becomes. If you can, just close your eyes, take three regular deep breaths to relax and try this simple visualisation exercise.

Picture yourself standing at the top of an escalator. Below, in a beautiful foyer, you can see an important social gathering. All of your friends are there. As you travel down the escalator you magically begin to shed all of your excess weight. By the time you reach the bottom you are at your ideal weight. Your are wearing clothes that show off this new you.

See this picture of yourself at your ideal weight. The weight you would choose to be if nothing stood in your way. Then form a firm, clear image of yourself at this ideal weight. Try to hold this mental image, clearly in your mind and ask yourself the following questions;

How do you feel about yourself?
How do you look?
What sort of clothes are you wearing?
What types of food would you eat?
How do the people around you relate to this
new ideal you?

Take a while to think on this image of the ideal you. This image will make you feel good about yourself, it will make you feel happier, more confident, more self-assured. This is how you should, and could feel all of the time - it is your natural state.

After feeling good about yourself, you will probably also experience a feeling of disappointment or frustration about the way you look now.

But, by answering the questions about how you felt and what you ate, your mind has given you clues on how to successfully lose weight. It has told you exactly the type of foods you need to eat, and how you need to feel in order to turn that ideal vision into reality. All we have to do now is to show you how to close this gap between the present you and the future you. Because, the very fact that you have the ability to picture the ideal you with imagination and emotion, means that you have it in your ability to make this vision a reality.

The No Diet - Diet will help you to bring your vision of the ideal you into reality. The techniques used need no special skills or training that you do not already possess. You do not need an iron will, it requires no special diet, there are no restricted foods and no rigid regimes. In fact it takes surprisingly little effort at all. There is a simple reason why losing weight can, and should be so easy.

The very latest scientific research on weight loss has concluded that the key to weight loss is in the mind, not in the stomach. The leading experts who have studied slimming - including many prominent doctors agree on this one thing. It is that the most important factor in successful long term weight loss is to actually change the slimmer's mental attitude to eating.

In her best-selling book No Sweat Fitness, Tania Alexander wrote "*...you don't physically have to do anything at all! All you need to do is start thinking thin and boosting your self image... for nothing holds more power over the body than the beliefs of the mind.*"

There is now a growing belief amongst the medical profession that you can change your body simply by changing your perception of it. The No Diet - Diet will teach you many of proven techniques that will enable you to adjust your beliefs, change your self concept and literally start to think yourself thinner!

If you follow the techniques outlined you will naturally and effortlessly start to lose weight - because you will simply stop thinking about, stop craving, and ultimately stop eating the foods that are wrong for you. By using these techniques on a consistent basis, you will never need to attempt to diet by using a traditional, structured weight loss programme again.

That is a promise.

Jim Brackin

www.jimbrackin.com

BEFORE WE START - A TIP

To regain control and make long term, lasting
changes to your life you only have to do three things
to ensure that you get the right result.

1. Use these techniques only when you are really
ready to make the change.

2. Follow the instructions and have faith
that they will, over time work.

3. Take all of the credit for the results you get.

Follow these three simple steps and
you'll find the No Diet, Diet path.

The new approach
to weight loss

If you are overweight, congratulations!

You are genetically superiour to 52% of all other human beings. The chances are that your metabolism is different to that of the other 48%. It allows you eat similar foods to them, but store more energy, in the form of fat, on your body. This gives you tremendous advantage in any society in which food is scarce or the food supply is intermittent. In times of famine, you would be the one with the best chance of survival.

Unfortunately, the Western World has not been known for its life threatening food shortages for over 150 years. Your genetic advantage cuts no ice in modern society. To add insult to genetic superiority, today being overweight is often viewed in a slightly different light.

I have tried many different ways to lose the visable signs of my genetic advantage. In over ten years of fighting an ever increasing waistline I have tried almost everything. I have restricted my eating to a limited number of fruits. I have spent hours carefully weighing out suggested menus.

Once in desperation I tried substituting brightly coloured drinks for natural foods!

All these endeavours have ended in failure - with little or no short term gain. All they left me with is a feeling of frustration. I was not in control of my own body. A feeling of resigned helplessness would hang over me like a cloud. I felt that weight loss was just not possible for me. It seemed that I was just destined to be fat, sorry, genetically superiour.

Having struggled with being overweight for a decade, I realised that, for some reason, the traditional methods of weight loss were not going to work for me. I found that any weight loss programme based on food restriction, deprivation, substitution or calorie counting was just destined to fail

However hard I tried to lose weight, my mental attitude was all wrong. While I felt a helpless bystander in the battle for my waistline, I was never going to win. To lose weight I had to change my attitude, which in turn would change my eating habits. Only then could I lose weight, and keep it off for life.

A few days after coming to this conclusion, by coincidence, I happened to watch an Oprah Winfrey show on the subject of weight loss. She said something that was to confirm my perception of weight loss. She said *"Diets don't work, you've got to get to the reason that lies behind overeating."*

This was something that I knew instinctively was correct, based on my personal experience. Now, having spent many years researching the subject I realised that there is also a growing body of physical evidence to support this view. With many confirmations coming from the latest research undertaken by the scientific community.

The University of London are currently revising their research on weightloss. In an ongoing study of effective and permanent weight reduction, they are testing a combination of positive psychology and diet control. This combination has been shown to be much more effective, in the long term, than the traditional diet control methods of weight loss.

A recent laboratory controlled study conducted at Littlemore Hospital, Oxford, England concluded that the effect of food restrictive, weight loss programmes were *"surprisingly ineffective as a means of achieving sustained weight loss."*

Most dieters, including myself, are typical of the behaviour patterns uncovered by their studies. Whenever I tried to lose weight by food restriction, one of two things always happened.

The first was that I would undertake a diet full of enthusiasm, only to find that within a short time, maybe a few days, a few weeks or just occasionally, a few months I got bored with the change in diet. I would then increasingly desire all of the foods I was not 'allowed' to eat. Eventually I reached a point where I would crack, and break my diet. After that I would drift back to my old eating pattern - the one that made me overweight in the first place - then, I just gave up. Another failure.

The other thing that happened was that the one time I did achieve my target weight, and mentally my diet was over, my old eating habits slowly started to return. This was actually much worse! I then proceeded to put back the weight I'd lost and much more besides.

These two behavioural patterns were highlighted as typical reactions to traditional weight loss programmes in the Littlemore study. I then began to hear of experiences of others, that followed exactly the same patterns. During the course of my research for this programme, many people have written to me and told of their experiences.

Kathleen Hockley, a dieter for over 40 years wrote to me explaining that *"Being overweight brings guilt and feelings of inferiority. I have been to every slimming club there has ever been. The lady at the front of the class tells us how self-indulgent we all are and how easy it will be not to give in any more to chocolate bars and bread and jam. I go to bed hungry. I eat things I don't like. Steamed puddings and roast potatoes are unknown quantities to me. I daren't eat what I want - I am tired of feeling guilty."*

Dawn Lloyd, who after a lifetime of struggling with her weight, wrote, *"I had tried everything in the past. Slim fast and all sorts of wonder pills, nothing had worked and I wasn't getting my hopes up. I just seemed to get fatter. The fatter I got the more I ate as comfort food."*

These feelings are typical of many hundreds of letters I have received. I realised that the feelings of guilt, frustration and helplessness that we often face alone are symptoms of a deep seated problem.

A Dietary & Nutritional Survey of British Adults commissioned by the Ministry of Agriculture, Fisheries & Food and the Department of Health, in 1993 found that 48% of women and 57% of men are overweight. Of them some 16% of women and 13% of men are clinically obese with over 20% of their body mass being fat.

DETERMINE YOUR CORRECT BODY WEIGHT

Being overweight as defined by the survey, was based on a measurement called the Body Mass Index. The Body Mass Index or BMI shows the relationship between your height and your weight and is the industry standard term used to define body size. It is measured using the following calculation; Your weight in Kgs divided by Your height in (Meters) squared.

For example your weight was 14st 9oz (93Kgs) and your height was 6ft 1ins (1.85m) the calculation would be 93 divided by 1.85x1.85 or 93- 3.42 giving a body mass indicator of 27.2. If, like me, maths is not your strong point, the chart on page 12 will give you a good indication of your BMI.

If you are typically underweight your BMI will be under 20. An ideal weight would produce a figure of between 20 and 25. With a BMI between 26 and 30 you would be considered as overweight and 30 or over would be defined as obese.

Your sex and frame size is already allowed for in this set of measurements - if, for example, you were at an ideal weight a smaller framed person would typically fall into the lower half of the scale (20-22), whereas a large male would be nearer the top end (24-25).

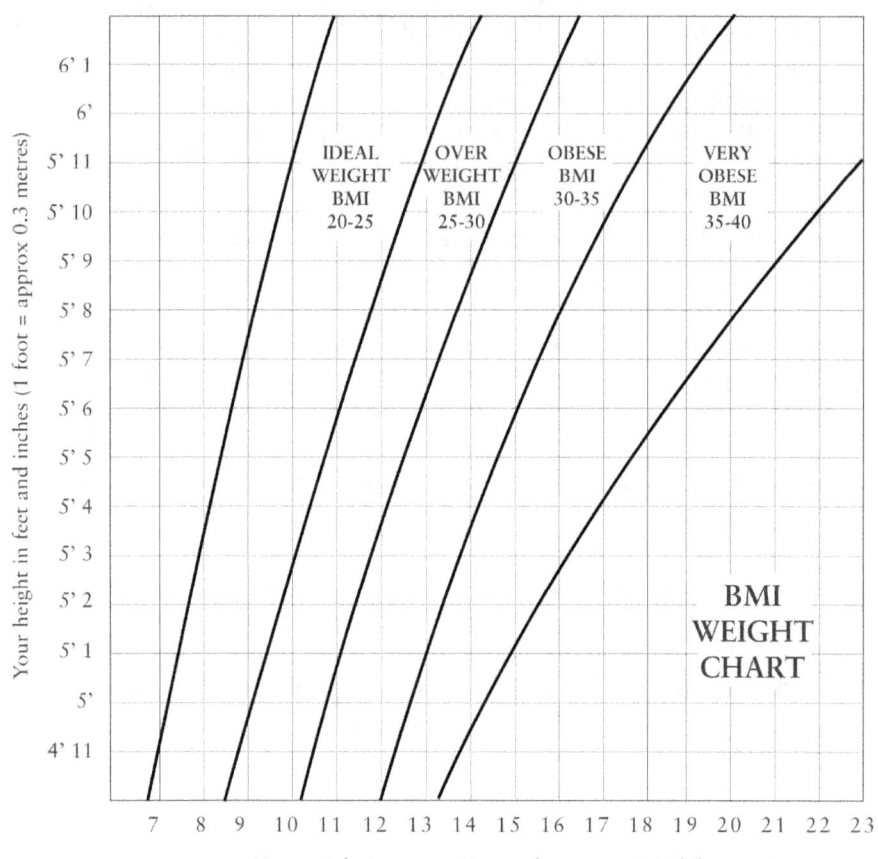

When deciding your ideal weight, use the BMI as an indicator, it is a good guide for real, healthy, normal people. By this definition every super model would be defined as underweight, they typically have a BMI of 18 or less.

WHY 98% OF ALL WEIGHT LOSS
PROGRAMMES FAIL

It's estimated that, in the UK at any one time over 58% of women and 33% of men are trying to lose weight. With a population of over 60 million people, that is well over 16 million people.

Janet Menzies, author of the DIY Diet, states *"The terrible truth about dieting is that 90% of all diets fail. Most professional nutritionists, diet researchers and many health writers have known this for some time."*

Rosemary Conley author of the Hip and Thigh Diet puts the figure even higher at 98%.

It seems it is an open secret that of those that are on a diet 92% will fail before reaching their target weight. Another 6% will actually reach their ideal weight only to put it all back on within two years - that leaves 2% of dieters who are successful. The definition of successful being someone who has kept to their target weight for over 3 or more years.

The Health and Diet Industry spends over £6 billion per year on advertising. It has over 16 million people participating, using its hundreds of different types of slimming products, reading over 340,000 slimming books per year.

The result of all of this effort and expenditure - just a 2% success rate!

Doesn't it strike you that there must be something wrong here?

Why do most people fail? From a medical point of view, we know that the vast majority of the weight loss programmes would work if followed. One the whole they are nutritious, well balanced and designed to reduce your weight - yet 98% still end in failure.

It is obvious to me that there must be some crucial factor missing from the existing methods of weight loss. Why else would the success rate be so low? On the evidence presented we must seriously question and re-think the way in which we approach the entire subject.

I've thought about this question for many years. I have read every book on slimming, nutrition, psychology, physiology and motivation I could, I have listened to tapes and have spent thousands of pounds on, and hours immersed in the subject of weight loss.

You can't but come to one very simple conclusion.

The reason that 98% of weight loss programmes fail is that they fail to pay attention to the one critical factor that controls your weight - and that's your mind. The way you think about yourself and the food you eat is the key determinant of your weight. To be slim you have think slim. To do this you should first change your mental attitudes towards food and your weight.

THE SCIENTIFIC EVIDENCE

The realisation that slimming is all in the mind was one of the findings made by the five scientists researching the effects of weight loss at Littlemore Hospital, Oxford. Dr

Clifford, and colleagues conducted a controlled study on behalf of the Medical Research Council, Wellcome Trust and the Mental Health Foundation.

During the research, they discovered that when we undertake a food restrictive weight loss programme, a side effect is that the brain is starved of serotonin - a chemical known to control the appetite. As a result of this reduction in the level of serotonin the brain naturally produces more to compensate. This is a typical defensive reaction to protect the body's food supply. But not only does it produce more serotonin, it typically produces an excess. It is this excess of serotonin that stimulates the dieter to increase their food intake. Which is exactly the opposite result to the one intended by dieting.

> Their study concluded that *"Humans have evolved powerful adaptive mechanisms for maintaining food intake. Trying to overcome these by voluntary food restriction is not only difficult, but may be counter productive in some individuals."*

This seems to be a logical, reliable, scientific explanation for what the 98% of us, attempting to lose weight, have experienced for years. If you consume less, you also remain hungry, which is counterproductive to sustaining a long term change in diet and weight.

Based on my own observations and experiences, I believe that if we do not consciously try to restrict our food intake we automatically over-ride the process that makes us produce excess serotonin.

That is why the techniques used in this programme never consciously attempt to restrict the food you eat. Any changes you decide to make to your diet are made at a subconscious level. Or are so small a change as to seem, in the short term, insignificant. Actually you will be encouraged to eat more than you do now, of the right kinds of food.

Losing weight does not equal feeling hungry or being totally deprived of your favourite foods. Exactly the opposite is often true. Each person's metabolic rate responds to the amount of food that they eat. Deprive yourself of food and the body's ability to burn fat is reduced. This is why food depravation has exactly the opposite effect to the one intended. It is better to eat more high bulk, low-fat and nutritious foods.

A good example of this was highlighten by an experiment conducted in America. A group of overweight volunteers were encouraged to eat whatever they wanted. With one condition. They had to eat 3lbs potatoes a day, before they ate anything else. Once they had eaten the potatotes they could indulge themselves to their hearts content, no food was off-limits.

Over a six month period all of the volunteers had lost between 12lbs and 25lbs in weight. Simply, by filling up on a low calorie, high bulk food they had supressed their desire for the high calorie, low bulk foods. The foods that made them overweight in the first place.

There are many ways to lose weight without feeling hungry. Many are discussed in this programme and because psychologically, you are never on a weight loss diet, your mind is not programmed to produce excess seratonin in the way it does with a food restrictive programme. That's why you will never feel hungry using these techniques - even though you are steadily losing weight.

To lose weight you must have the right mental attitude. This is where your previous experiences are so important because, if you have already tried and failed to lose weight, you already know that having the desire and motivation alone is not sufficient to succeed. What you also need are the techniques and methodology to achieve your ideal weight. Most of us have a burning desire to lose weight without ever planning or thinking about how we are going to achieve it.

We already know that 98% of externally imposed weight loss programmes will not work on their own. I believe the reason is simple. It is because they attempt change our existing and preferred eating pattern without also changing our thinking.

The more extreme this attempted change is, the more likely the weight loss programme is to fail - and quickly. Best estimates indicate that over 50% fail in the first three to five days of being started. This suggests that the more dramatic the enforced change in diet, the stronger your desire to return to your original diet.

Logically the smaller the change in your diet, the less desire you have to revert back. This is one of the key principles behind the No Diet-Diet Weight Loss Programme. A small change now can make a big difference in a year.

Imagine what two or three small changes would make.

You are an individual. You are unique, your experiences, your viewpoints, your knowledge, your dress sense, your preferences, and eating habits are yours and yours alone. These are the things have made you what you are, surely they should play an important part in you attempts to lose weight.

Yet, most food based weight loss programmes impose their own restrictions on what you can and cannot eat. They do not see you as an individual. Your unique preferences, circumstances and eating patterns just do not feature in the equation. Any system that denies your choice as an individual is much more likely to be rejected.

You are the only person who can decide what you eat, and when you eat it. It is your choice and your responsibility. You are in control, and need to re-evaluate a strongly held belief. To successfully lose weight you must dispel the myth that weight loss is based on the need to count calories, deprive yourself of certain foods, or artificially change your eating habits - it's not.

The food we eat is only half of the answer. Unless we take into account our mental attitude towards the foods we eat, we will continue to fail ito lose weight in our millions. This type of traditional food focus weight loss programme is almost impossible to sustain in the long term - as the 98% failure rate suggests!

The focus of maintainable, long term weight loss, should be on what motivates us to eat what we eat. Change the way you think and you change the way you eat. In reality, attitude is the single most critical determinant of your weight; for attitude determines your eating habits - so much so that even your choice of studying this programme is making a positive commitment to weight loss.

The way you think and the beliefs you have can effect your body in surprising ways. Researchers at the New England Medical Centre discovered in tests that between 70% and 90% of their patients could reduce the effects of their illnesses. They were also able to reduce their recovery times, simply by adopting a positive mental attitude toward the illness. Dr H. Benson, who led the research commented *"Belief in a good outcome can have formidable restorative power."*

What motivates us to eat what we eat is our self-concept, how we think about ourselves. We, as intelligent, thinking human beings are totally responsible for all of our actions. It's our thoughts, attitudes and mental health that determine our needs, desires and cravings.

We must accept that our weight is governed by the actions we have taken in our lives. The one, and only, thing you have total control over is what you think. Only you can decide what thoughts you have inside your head. You have chosen the foods you eat, dictated by behaviour patterns that you have consciously or unconsciously programmed into your subconscious.

You are, therefore, totally responsible for the way you look and feel today.

Slimming Magazine wrote "*Your first step to happiness is to recognise this truth: that if you are overweight, in the wrong job, frustrated, it truly isn't anybody else's fault. Not ever. Your happiness and fulfilment are your responsibility.*"

A psychologist would tell you that weight closely mirrors your present self-concept. If you are overweight it is for a reason. Unless you are one of the unfortunate 0.1% of people who are overweight because of a medical problem, you eat more that you need to sustain your existing lifestyle. Find the reason (or reasons) why and you can change them. If you change your self-concept you can automatically change your weight. If you can change the way that you think about food, you can change your body's reaction to it and need for it.

This is a really exciting concept - you can actually think yourself slimmer.

THE TRUE MEANING OF DIET

The relationship between mental attitude and weight is not a new concept, in fact, it's been known for centuries. It is where the word Diet comes from. Diet is derived from the Latin "*Diaeta*" and is defined in the Oxford English Dictionary as a "*Way of living or thinking*". In the original sense of the word a Diet is a holistic approach, a mental process, a method of using your thoughts to control your life.

Ellington Darden Phd, author of The Nautilus Diet, wrote "*Most people think of a diet as a temporary way of*

WHAT DO YOU SEE IN THE MAIN PICTURE, AN OLD WOMAN OR A YOUNG GIRL?

Both are clearly visible in the picture, The one that you see depends not on reality, but your own perception of it. Think of this as a metaphor for your own self image. Your reality, like your potential is unlimited, it is only your existing self-limiting beliefs that hold you back.

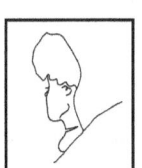

The old
woman

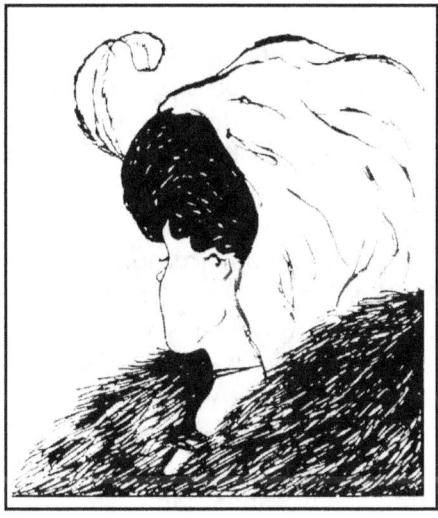

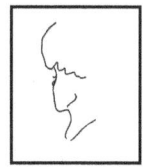

The
young girl

restricting food to lose weight. Once they've lost the desired weight, the diet is discarded and old eating habits are resumed...a diet is not a temporary route to a short-term goal. A diet is a blueprint for your life."

We, in our modern desire to lose weight quickly, seem to have forgotten this ancient truth. It is our thoughts, our hopes, our self-concept, our values and our goals that determine and direct our lives - what we think determines what we eat. You must think slim before you can be slim.

In its original meaning, Diet was not a word for some kind of externally imposed method of food restriction to achieve weight loss. Diet is a word that describes the method of directing your life from within using the power of your thoughts.

Only in recent times has the word diet come to be associated with a *"Prescribed course of food, restricted in kind or quality"*. That is why, when I describe other so-called diets, I use the term weight loss programmes - they are not, in the true sense of the word, diets.

There is another good reason for this distinction. Psychologically this distinction also helps you to clearly differentiate between any failures you associate with *"dieting"*, in its' corrupted sense. It enables your to look forward to future success.

Let's start to diet successfully, in the sense of its original meaning, right now. Let's start the process of thinking slim.

Developing the techniques of thinking slim is the fundamental difference between the No Diet - Diet and the other weight loss programmes you may have tried and that have left you disappointed. You will find no recipes, no plans or regimes in this programme.

That is because the secret of weight loss is not just about an artificially imposed restriction of food. Everyone who has practised the techniques of the No Diet-Diet on a regular basis has lost weight without consciously restricting certain foods.

I personally have not cut any food from my normal diet. I have however, changed my attitude towards food so that now I chose to eat certain foods often more than others.

Based on the strategies that we will share in this programme, you will be able to make more informed choices that are based on your lifestyle and personal circumstances. You are free to use any of the strategies, in any what that you see fit.

You are a responsible person, who is in total control of your eating habits. You will make the right choices for your own needs. But whatever you do you are totally responsible for the way you look, and will look in the future.

I, like many who have used this programme still drink real ale, wine and spirits. I still love ice cream. I occasionally indulge my desire for chocolate.

I still eat many of the foods that used to make me overweight. Yet using the techniques in this programme, I still was able to lose two stone in six months. I was able to achieve my ideal weight by changing my attitude toward food. I have maintained that ideal weight ever since and am totally confident of doing so for the rest of my life.

CHANGE YOUR ATTITUDE, AND CHANGE YOUR WEIGHT

This dramatic turnaround has come about simply because I have changed my attitude to the food I eat. I have not changed the food, but I have changed my eating patterns. Now my self-concept is permanently changed. I think like a slim person; I feel like a slim person and I act like a slim person. My body behaves in a manner consistent with this self-concept. Subsequently I desire less of the foods that make me increase weight, and genuinely enjoy more of the foods that help me lose it. It really is that simple and this is how it works.

Your self-concept is made up of the sum total of your self image, your self esteem and your self-confidence. One of the key objectives of this programme is to show you a number of practical techniques that will raise your levels of self-image, self esteem and self-confidence.

All three are important factors in helping you to lose weight. If you worry about, and have tried unsuccessfully to lose weight, you will have a low self-concept about your ability in this area. Being overweight affects your self-image.

As you have probably already experienced, no one has ever felt good about themselves when they have felt that they are overweight. They feel negative about buying clothes, uncomfortable about the thought of a trip to the local swimming pool, guilty about what they eat, nervous about being the focus of attention. They are constantly consumed by their weight. This simply re-inforces the negative emotions already attached to their self-concept.

This was highlighted in a letter I received recently from Denise Tilbury, who in her own words had been "a little dumpy" from her teenage years. She wrote, *"My self-image was low for many years, and being overweight and unable to control my eating added to the lack of self esteem. For several years, these were the problems that occupied my mind from the moment I woke up each day."*

As Denise had experienced, if you are conscious of being overweight this will tend to occupy your thoughts. By worrying about it you produce negative thoughts which undermine your self-image , which in turn will affect your self esteem. Because of this your self-confidence suffers. This often results in feelings of helplessness, frustration and lack of control. These are physically manifested in habit, comfort or binge eating. All of which result in you eating more of the foods you know will make you put on weight, which of course is exactly what happens, and the whole process becomes a vicious circle.

You become trapped in a circle of negative re-enforcement, which is manifested by feeling of helplessness, frustration and resignation. But, this circle can easily be broken if you know how.

If you raise your self-concept, and change the way you think about yourself, you can programme your body to act and behave in a manner consistent with this 'raised' awareness - this alone is enough to encourage you lose weight.

To raise your self-concept is surprisingly easy. It takes just a few minutes a day over a period of between two weeks and a month. As your self-concept changes you will also see the weight just dissolving away. You will be amazed that you're actually losing weight, because you will just not feel as if you are on a diet!

THINK YOURSELF THINNER - THE EXPERTS VIEW

My research into this exciting method of weight control has revealed that many of the leading diet and nutrition experts believe that the power of the mind has a profound influence on weight loss.

In her book Lose 7lbs in 7 days, Dr Miriam Stoppard observed *"We have to acquire a new personal psychology of eating - not an easy job when so many bad habits have to be unlearned."*

Dr Deepak Chopra who was described by Vogue as the medical mentor of the 90's, wrote in his best-selling book Ageless Body, Timeless Mind *"The line between biology and psychology can't really be drawn with any great certainty ... the mind influences every cell in our body ... if you want to change your body, change your awareness first ...you can change your body simply by changing your perception."*

Slimming Magazine published a book called The 30 Day Formula which stated *"It is this low self esteem that makes it so difficult for many to keep to a diet and lose weight. This fundamental feeling of unworthiness and very low self-regard has to be explored - and then exploded."*

Psychologist Paul Goldin, an expert in the field of weight control, believes that *"Diet advice that fails to alter an individual's food belief systems is just meaningless."*

The importance of your thoughts in the process of weight loss are often touched upon in slimming books. Many recognise its importance, then fail to expand on the subject in any detail. Instead they take the obvious, safe and often commercially lucrative route by printing pages upon pages of recipes to follow.

The No Diet-Diet is very different, it provides you with the very best techniques and strategies to change your mindset, perceptions and behaviours, and to put your new no diet mentality into practice right away.

IS THE RECTANGLE ON THE RIGHT LARGER THAN THE RECTANGLE ON THE LEFT?

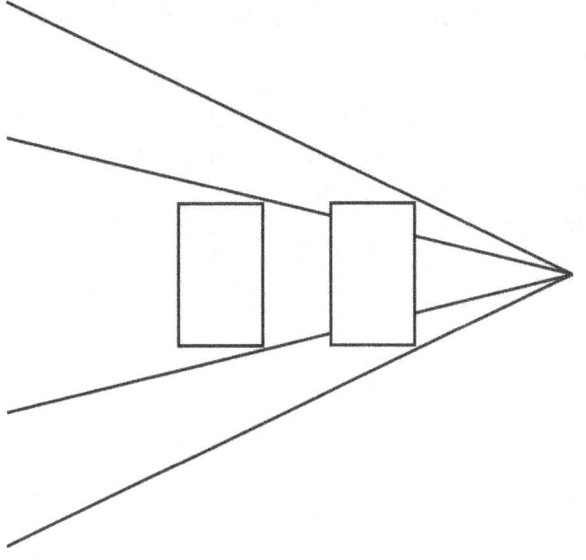

No. They are both the same size. It is the perspective that fools the eye into believing that the right hand rectangle is larger. Don't allow outside inflences to dictate your size.

Appreciate yourself - you're unbelievable

Next it is important for you to understand how your mind and body work, and how they interact. Understanding this intimate relationship is a crucial first step to thinking yourself slimmer. Although you do not need to understand how any of the techniques in this book work for them to be successful, if you understand the theory as well as the practice, this additional knowledge will move you more quickly towards your desired weight loss.

Peter Russell, author of The Brain Book, wrote

"Within our heads lies one of the most complex systems in the known universe. Its power and versatility far surpass that of any manmade computer, and no human being has ever come anywhere near to using its full potential."

YOUR BRAIN IS FANTASTIC

The brain is very sensitive to it's surroundings. There are even some that can detect the smallest differences in sound, light, smell and touch. They organise and regulate the body's life functions, learn from experience, communicate using language. These brains are so sensitive that they can detect changes in magnetic and electromagnetic fields. They can detect ultraviolet light and analyse the polarisation of sunlight and use this analysis to tell direction. They can keep an accurate track of time even in the dead of night.

These skills are amazing, especially when you consider that the brain I am describing is not the brain of a human being but, that of a honey bee. It is no bigger than a grain of sand and contains about 900 brain cells called neurons.

Your brain contains over ten billion neurons. Each of those neurons is connected to ten thousand other neurons. It has been estimated that the world's entire telephone system is not as complex as one single ounce of your brain. Your mind's complexity is totally staggering.

It is known that your brain has the capacity to store every thought or experience you have in your lifetime. The reason that we forget things is not that we do not remember them, it is because we have difficulty accessing the information, unless it has an emotional trigger attached to it. The emotion links a chemical trigger to the memory that makes it easy to recall.

That is why you can remember in minute detail some key events that happened years ago, but may forget what you were doing this time last month. The ability to remember is totally determined by the emotional attachment you attribute to the experience.

How your mind works

It was Dr. Paul MacLean who first proposed the view that the human brain is in reality three brains, each of which has been superimposed over the earlier one - which is exactly how they look when the brain is seen in cross-section.

The first, oldest and most primitive is the reptilian brain. The reptilian brain is totally driven by instinct and is the home of your innermost feelings.

Second is the limbic, or mammalian brain. This encircles the reptilian brain. It controls the body's autonomic nervous system. It is the part that regulates, amongst other things, eating, drinking, hunger, walking, sleeping, body temperature, blood pressure, and heat rate. This is the part of the brain that is the core of your emotions.

The third and most recent is the neocortex, which accounts for over 80% of the total matter in the brain. It is this that distinguishes us from the other higher mammals - the neocortex in humans is large in relation to our body size. The neocortex is what makes us act and think as human beings. It allows us to think, perceive, speak and rationalise.

Apart from the size and potential of our brain, we differ in one very important aspect from almost every other creature, our neocortex gives us the faculty of self-consciousness. We are aware of ourselves as conscious beings, and have the ability to draw on our previous experiences and apply them to new situations even though they are totally unrelated.

In fact, one definition of intelligence is not how much we know, but how we react in a situation when we don't know what to do.

WHAT YOU THINK IS WHAT YOU ARE

It's not surprising then that this fantastic organ exerts a very powerful influence on the body. Every thought you have starts its life when a brain cell releases a chemical, which via the synaptic gap (the gap between the brain cells) is transferred to the next cell. If the thought is a strong one this starts a chemical chain reaction, branching out to millions of other cells around the brain.

Every thought you have is a chemical chain reaction - a very real, measurable and physical thing. There are over 100,000 of these chemical reactions taking place in your brain every second and they have a profound effect on every cell in your body. Your body physically responds to every one of your thoughts.

Many doctors now believe that 70% of illnesses can be directly traced back to some form of mental imbalance - stress being the major imbalance. If the mind is unwell the body will show this as a physical manifestation. Your mental state is a key determinant of your health, so be very careful what you think about because negative thoughts which produce stress and anxiety can, and actually do, trigger certain illnesses.

The reverse is also true.

There is a well documented case in the U.S. of a woman who treated terminally ill cancer patients - without drugs, just by using the power of suggestion. Her method involved making her patients visualise their white blood cells as piranha fish, which were thriving and rapidly feeding on the tumours that were visualised as hamburger meat.

This might seem a stange treatment, but within just a few weeks the white cell blood counts of the patients had unexpectedly increased in number; this defied any normal medical explanation. The cancerous tumours had also reduced in size.

A medical study conducted by Stanford psychiatrist David Spiegal clearly demonstrated that changing a patients beliefs could offset the effects of breast cancer.

He took 86 women with breast cancer beyond the help of normal treatment and gave half of them lessons in self-hypnosis, combined with weekly psychotherapy. He monitored their progress for ten years. The group that received the therapy survived on average twice as long as the control group.

This has been reflected by other similar findings. A 1987 study from Yale reported that women with low self-concepts were more likely to develop breast cancer. The same has been found to be true of asthma, and rheumatoid arthritis.

WHICH OF THE FIGURES IS THE WIDER?

Although the figure on the right looks wider, they are in fact exactly the same. Like the figures below your perceptions of are not always based on fact or reality they are often based on old or inaccurate assumptions. Change the assumptions and you can change the way you see yourself.

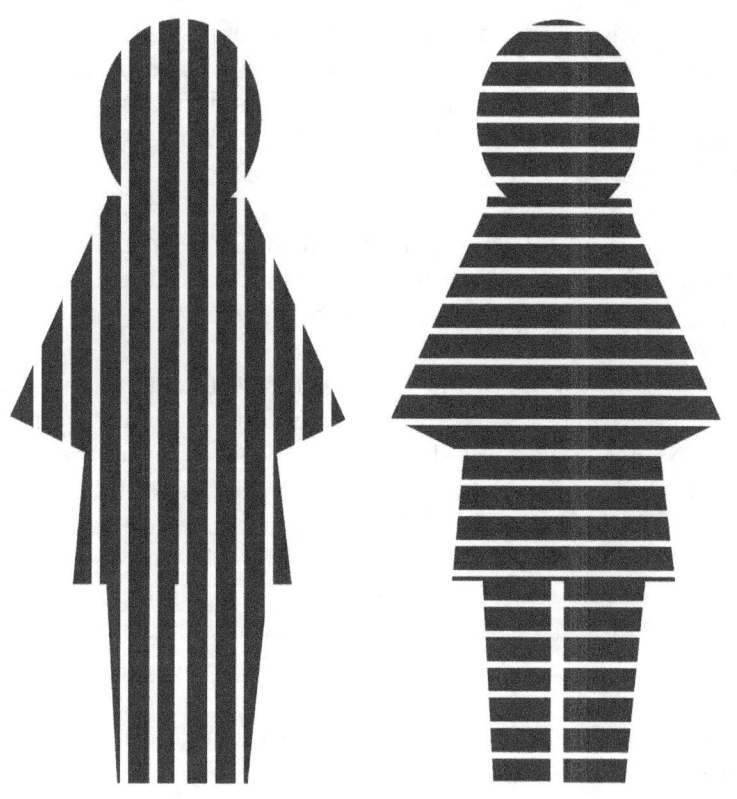

It has also been shown that patients who are given a placebo - a medicine that has no active drug to cure the patient's condition - often react as if the normal treatment has been given.

It works because the patients believe that they are being treated for their condition. They believe the treatment is working and their bodies start to react as if it really was - even though the 'cure' is totally in their minds. They actually treat themselves.

In one landmark study a group of patients with bleeding ulcers were divided into two groups.

Both groups were given a placebo. One group were told that they were being given a drug that *"was absolutely guaranteed to provide relief."* The other group were told that they were being given *"an experimental drug, but little was known about it's side effects."* Of the first group 70% experienced a major relief of their symptoms, while only 25% of the second group had a similar result.

The 'treatment' was the same for both groups. Yet the group with high levels of expectation and belief were nearly 300% more likely to find relief.

That is how a placebo works, it contains no drugs to improve the user's condition - it relies on the patient's expectation and belief. The patient's body actually manufactures the right chemicals to treat the condition. And to the degree that the patient believes that the treatment will have an positive effect - it does.

CH-CH-CHANGES

Your body is an amazing organism, which has been developing and changing ever since you were conceived. It is still changing at a surprising rate. Every breath you exhale expels countless thousands of atoms that were previously part of your heart, liver, kidneys, and other parts of your body.

You are endlessly changing. Every month your skin is replaced. Every six weeks your liver is replaced. Every three months your skeleton is replaced. In just twelve months your body actually replaces 98% of the physical matter it consists of. So, in a years time you really will be physically a different person.

It is this dynamic change is what makes us so durable.
It enables us to constantly repair our bodies - unlike objects that are static which naturally atrophy and degenerate. Metals rust, mountains erode, plastic compounds bio-degrade, they can do nothing else - they cannot adapt to their circumstances. Whereas you can.

You now know, your physical body will be totally different in twelve months' time. However, the one thing that keeps you the way you are, the blueprint of what you will be is determined by your innermost thoughts, your self-concept. This blueprint is then actioned through the body's DNA. It is your DNA determines your genetic pattern. Although originally your DNA is inherited from your parents, the information it contains is not beyond your ability to change. In studies conducted in America, DNA has been shown to react in different ways dependant on mental state. The way you think can have a subtle effect on your genetic makeup.

Your self-concept the sum total of your beliefs, your expectations, your values and your self esteem. It's the combination of these thoughts which are imprinted on your limbic system that is your subconscious mind, that determine how you will physically look, now and in the future.

Your subconscious or limbic system is the part of your brain that deals with the running of the body. Without conscious thought it controls all your life functions - your heart-rate, breathing, temperature, posture, size, movement, in fact everything that makes you. And it's all automatic, you don't have to do a thing.

The function of the subconscious dictates that it works in the present, or to use a phrase you may have heard athletes use *"in the now"*. For example, if you were crossing a road and become aware of a car speeding towards you, as soon as your conscious mind became alerted to the danger, the subconscious mind takes over. It's only goal is to get you out of danger. You don't consciously decide which foot to move, or whether you are going to move forward or backwards. Your subconscious takes over and you 'instinctively' get out of the way.

This is a really important point. Because it does not analyse situations the subconscious totally believes everything you tell it - whether what you tell it is real or imaginary, true or false. It has to do this because your life might depend on it.

You will have experienced this for yourself - how often have you been engrossed in a film when something scary or unexpected happens? You are startled, or you jump up, just as if the situation was actually happening to you. Of course a fraction of a second later, after you have jumped out of you skin, you remind yourself that it's just a movie - and relax again.

But for that split second, your subconscious was fully alert, in that split second your heart rate was raised, your muscles tensed, adrenaline was pumped into your system, ready for you to flee this celluloid assailant.

The subconscious could not distinguish between fact and fiction, it just faithfully reacted to your suggestion.

We can use the way your subconscious works to our own advantage. We know that the subconscious will always make us behave in a manner consistent with our self-concept, so it follows that just by changing the way you think about dieting, you will change the way you behave.

The quickest most effective way to do this is by using positive affirmations.

Think yourself slimmer!

Affirmations are a highly effective way to programme our subconscious to act in a manner consistent with our desires. They are a form of mental conditioning used by many top achievers to increase their performance.

All top athletes and sports people have affirmations and use them constantly - often in conjunction with some form of positive visualisation, which is explained in more detail in lesson six. Affirmations are used because they are very, very effective and have been described as the single most important factor in improved achievement. Often athletes are physically evenly matched and the only difference between them is their will to win. Anything that makes that will stronger could make the crucial difference between being an average athlete or a great one. Less than 0.2 of a second seperated the gold medalist from fourth place in the final of the mens 100 meters at the Barcelona Olympics. In percentage terms that is less than a 0.5% difference.

We can use affirmations to increase our willpower to help us lose weight. When I have taught affirmation and visualisation techniques to others, they have typically shown improvements of between 5 and 10%. But, the effects do not have to be immediate, or large to have a dramatic effect. That is not the function of affirmations, they are used primarily to tip the balance in our favour.

Affirmations give us a small advantage, typically just 1% or 2% would make the necessary difference. If the average person were to lose just 1% of their body weight every month, they would be 18lbs lighter in a years time!

Affirmations also have another use, they help to keep your self image consistent with your weight loss. One of the reasons that people reach their goal weight only to put the weight back on is that their new weight and their self image are inconsistent. There is a classic example of this inbalance shown in the case of Micheal Hebranko.

You might of heard his name, you probably remember his five minutes of fame. In 1995 the front of his house had to be demolished to get him to hospital. As Micheal was lifted from his home by a forklift truck, strapped to a sling normally used to carry dolphins and small whales this spectacle was broadcast across the world and watched by millions. At that time Micheal weighed 57 stone.

This was light by his standards, Micheal used to weigh 71 stone. He then slimmed to a trim 14 stone in just two years and made it into the Guinness Book of Records. He had recorded the greatest weight-loss ever measured. But it was not to last, he can remember the exact moment when he started to overeat and the reason why, *"I took care of the physical problem but not the emotional one, I didn't want to open up Pandora's box."* Despite his amazing weight-loss his self image was still that of an overweight man. This imbalance had to be corrected one way or another and it was, he reverted to his old habit patterns and started to regain the weight he had lost. He ate his way back up to 57 stone and T.V. stardom.

We can all learn from Micheal Hebranko, and use affirmations to keep our self image consistent with our desired physical reality.

The immediate use for the affirmation techniques below is to help you lose 1% to 2% of your bodyweight per month. Many people have. Affirmations are one of the most powerful techniques that you can use to think yourself thinner.

If you use just this one technique on a regular basis, and I would recommend at least once a day, you will quickly start to notice it's effect. Positive affirmations will start to overwrite all of the negative emotions that you have come to associate with slimming over the years. The more you use affirmations the quicker this over-writing will occur. Eventually the affirmation will become part of your behaviour, part of your positive self-image.

THREE LITTLE WORDS - ONE BIG CHANGE

Before I explain the key rules for affirmations, I would like you to try the following affirmation. It's a general "feel good" affirmation that will help increase your self esteem, which is lowered every time you have been reminded about being overweight and have felt guilty, frustrated or resigned to the fact that you are not in control.

If you can, look at yourself in a mirror. Repeat five times, out loud, with feeling and conviction:

> *"I like myself"*
> *"I like myself"*
> *"I like myself"*
> *"I like myself"*
> *"I like myself"*

If you can't bring yourself to say *"I like myself"* out loud then think it clearly and positively.

The first time you say it, you'll probably feel strange, maybe even a little embarrassed, or perhaps it gave you a little tingle down your spine. These are usual reactions, and happen because the affirmation contradicts your existing self-image.

It is easy for people who are embarrassed or challenged by this technique to dismiss affirmations as "silly" or "psycho-babble". This is not the view held in modern psychology. Brian Tracy author of a series of psychology programmes wrote, *"The core of self-concept is high self-esteem. A person with high self-esteem likes himself. How much you like yourself is the key determinant of your performance and your effectiveness in everything you do."* I know that the affirmation may sound strange, it did for me at first, but I urge you to try it and discover the difference it makes.

But, by the time you have said *"I like myself"* five times with feeling you just can't help but smile, to feel happy, to feel good about yourself. This simple act of saying *"I like myself, I like myself, I like myself, I like myself, I like myself"* has already started to re-programme your existing self-concept.

When I teach this positive affirmation technique, it's usually at this point that someone asks me if this is not just encouraging vanity. It's a good question. There is a very important distinction to be made between liking yourself and vanity.

To learn to appreciate your finer qualities is not being vain. Vanity is a term used to describe someone who delights in attracting the admiration of others - this is very different to appreciating yourself for what you are.

Until you genuinely like yourself, how can you expect others to like you? It has even been said by psychologists that you cannot like someone else more than you like yourself. Your relationships with every other person you know will be directly determined by your self-concept, by how much you like yourself.

You will have witnessed this yourself, people who are always depressed, unhappy or grumbling about life rarely have a large circle of friends. And the few friends they have tend to be just like them. Like attracts like.

Yet people with high self-concept are happy, responsible, likeable people, and because of this they are more fun to be with. People who are fun to be with tend to have large circles of friends.

"*I like myself*" is a general affirmation that makes you feel good about yourself. And feeling good about yourself is vitally important, because most people who are overweight do not feel good about themselves. They feel down because they look too big, they feel depressed because they are guilty about the food they eat, they feel negative because they are not in control of their weight.

BANISH NEGATIVE THOUGHTS

These negative feelings filter down to the unconscious. Consistently programming the unconscious with negative thoughts, creates self-limiting beliefs like, "*I can't lose weight, I'm not in control, it's my metabolism, it's genetic, it's not my fault, I'm resigned to be fat, diets don't work for me*" - all of these thoughts become firmly rooted in the self-concept over many years.

Then, when they do fail at losing weight, as they have programmed themselves to do, this simply confirms and strengthens their existing negative beliefs - it becomes a self-fulfilling prophecy.

Sylvia Simnett summed up this cause-and-effect perfectly over ten years ago in her booklet Slimmers in Extremis when she observed;

"*Most conventional slimmers think that will-power consists of an unbending attitude towards fat-producing foods. They grit their teeth and proclaim; I will not eat any more pastries. I will not eat chocolate between meals. All the time they are feeding their subconscious minds with negative ideas.*"

The simple act of using a positive affirmation and saying "*I like myself*" will start to redress the balance. If you say it, or think it on a regular basis, you will just be amazed at how good it will make you feel. It immediately starts to overwrite all of those negative emotions lodged in the self-concept. You will start to stand a little taller, feel a bit better and will have subtly changed your attitude to food - because if you feel good about yourself you'll want to lose weight.

There are many other affirmations that you should use on a regular basis. Two that are specifically designed to help you think slimmer are:

"*I only eat healthy foods*".

I advised a relative to use this "weight loss" affirmation on a regular basis, especially before meals. He lost over three stone in as many months.

"*I only eat healthy foods*" works surprisingly well as "weight loss" affirmation, because it re-programmes your unconscious to think carefully about the foods that you eat. Because it is non-specific it also gives your unconscious the freedom to choose the foods that will achieve, for you, a slim, trim figure.

If you use this "weight loss" affirmation on a regular basis, you will find that you will stop craving certain foods - always the ones that are keeping your weight on. It will just not occur to you to eat them, so you will either eat them less or not at all. It is not uncommon for chocaholics to totally lose the desire to eat chocolate after using this affirmation.

One told me *"I have been eating chocolate all my life, usually two or three bars a day...now I hardly touch the stuff, I find I do not really like the taste."*

This is typical of the effect a positive affirmation has - you start losing weight, as a direct consequence of changing your eating habits, but you do not feel like you are on a diet - because you're not. You are just eating foods that are consistent with your new self-concept. This is a very important distinction to make.

Eating is also about control - who controls when and how you eat and what you eat. Most overweight people have relinquished that control. They disassociate themselves from the decision to eat, by using terms like, *"I can't help it"*, *"I lost control"* or *"It was irrestable"*. They eat for comfort, or out of habit, or for social reasons but, rarely because they are actually hungry.

To lose weight you need to regain control of your eating patterns. There is a "control" affirmation that will help you to do this, it is an important affirmation that like many of the affirmations used in this book is valuable beyond the need to lose weight. It is,

> *"I'm am in control of my body, because I am totally responsible for everything that I eat".*

There is a shortened version of this that you should use on a regular basis.

> *"I'm in control, I am totally responsible for what I eat".*

Repeat this affirmation five times and while you do visualise yourself physically taking control of your eating habit. Visualise yourself refusing that Belgian Bun at lunch time or resisting the temptation of buying chocolate the supermarket checkout or turning down that extra helping of dessert at your favourite restaurant. Whatever situation you visualise it must show you taking control and choosing not to have the thing that will make you fat.

Now repeat five times,

"I'm in control, I am responsible for what I eat".
"I'm in control, I am responsible for what I eat".
"I'm in control, I am responsible for what I eat".
"I'm in control, I am responsible for what I eat".
"I'm in control, I am responsible for what I eat".

You should use these "control" affirmations on a regular basis in conjunction with visualising yourself in that position of control. When I started using this method I used to have a Belgian Bun (yes, that example above was drawn from personal experience!) every lunch time. After a few days I found that they just stopped looking so appealing. The sugar coating, which previously looked so good, started to look rater sickly. Consequently I stopped buying them, turning instead to the much healthier alternative of fresh fruit. Now when I look at the cakes on offer at the bakery, I just can't believe that I actually bought those sugar-coated weight enhancers and enjoyed eating them. I think my self esteem must have been pretty low at that time!

By now, you will have noticed that there is some degree of repetition in this chapter and indeed that is echoed throughout the book. There are two very good reasons for this.

Firstly, many of the areas discussed are inter-related and dependant upon each other. Within this programme they are organised into a logical order, which builds up to the complete picture, but in order to put some of the ideas into context it is necessary for them to overlap in certain areas.

The second, and more important reason, is that repetition is the mother of skill. Every skill you have was acquired by learning its principles and practising them until they are perfect. There is a great truth in the saying practice makes perfect. For example; you learn the theory of a tennis serve, then learn the muscle movements associated with it and then you repeat them. Practising the movements thousands of times, gradually improving the technique, until it becomes second nature.

Learning a mental skill is exactly the same, the more you repeat it the better you get.

Now, why not repeat the six new "control" affirmations below. Use them on a regular basis and you will always be in control of what you eat and when you eat it.

> *"I am totally responsible for when I eat."*.
> *"I am totally responsible for how I look"*.
> *"I am in control of my body"*.
> *"I am responsible for everything in my life"*.
> *"I am aware of my needs, and I'm in control"*.
> *"I lose weight easily"*.

Having been shown the affirmations that I have found most effective, you can make them even more powerful if you personalise them to your own tastes and circumstances. Now, let me share with you how to create your own powerful affirmations.

HOW AFFIRMATIONS WORK.

Earlier we learned that the way you think about yourself dictates how you look and feel. We also learned that it is the limbic part of the brain that controls this influence over the body, and that the limbic part of the brain is the centre of your subconscious. We know that the subconscious cannot differentiate between a real or an imaginary feeling. We know that anything you think about and believe in with emotion will be accepted as a truth by your subconscious.

By using the right affirmations you can fool it into thinking that you are slim, and it will automatically set about bringing that vision into reality. The more you use positive affirmations to overwrite your existing self-concept the quicker and easier it will be for you to diet. It really is that simple.

Once you start re-programming your subconscious it will automatically begin to adjust your eating patterns in a manner consistent with your new slim self-concept.

You will find that you will start to crave certain foods less, eat less and cut some foods out of your diet altogether. Perhaps you will engage in more exercise. The point is, that whatever happens will be self selecting. It will be a diet unique to you, and your circumstances because it has come from within - it is not imposed from outside. It will be well balanced, nutritious and sustainable but, because no food is off limits, there will be no cravings, and no guilt.

The only difference you will notice is that you'll feel better about yourself, you will feel more positive because you are in control of your body and, of course, when you weigh yourself, you will be lighter.

When I first started using positive affirmations, I noticed some remarkable changes in my thinking and eating patterns. Over a four week period I had stopped eating between meals. I ceased to enjoy sugar in coffee. I found that I preferred lemon in tea instead of milk. I reduced my consumption of hard cheese by 70% and I had developed a real craving for fresh fruit salad in the mornings!

Over that four week period I also lost 8 pounds in weight. This did a great deal to reinforce my belief in all of those positive affirmations. I also never felt hungry. I never felt as if I was depriving myself of food. I never felt as if I was restricting my diet - and I still don't.

So, say out loud, think or write down those positive affirmations

"I like myself".
"I only eat foods consistent with a slim, trim figure".
"I only eat healthy foods".
"I am in control, I am totally responsible for what I eat.".
"I am totally responsible for when I eat.".
"I am totally responsible for how I look".
"I am in control of my body".

"I am responsible for the direction of my life".
"I am aware of my needs, and I'm in control".
"I lose weight easily".

MAKE UP YOUR OWN AFFIRMATIONS

Before I give you some more very effective affirmations, there are two important rules to consider, which are particularly useful if you want to make up your own affirmations. I strongly suggest that you do this, because the more personal the affirmations are, the better they will work for you.

Rule one, is that you can use affirmations at any time in the day, and the more you use them the quicker you will re-programme your new slimmer thinking habit patterns. By the law of cause and effect the quicker you put your affirmations into practice the quicker you will start to lose weight naturally and easily.

Thinking your affirmations is nearly as powerful as saying them - and a much better option if you are in a public place!

There are two times during the day when your unconscious mind is particularly receptive to the power of suggestion. The first is during the first hour of the day. Called the "Golden Hour" by Earl Nightingale, author of Think and Grow Rich, this hour is the very best time to use affirmations to improve your self-concept. The last hour of the day is also an excellent time to use affirmations to re-affirm your desired habit patterns.

WHICH OF THE INNER CIRCLES IS THE LARGEST?

*Think of this a visual demonstration for positive thinking.
When you are feeling negative and you allow you problems
to grow in size (left) your influence seems much smaller, but
with a positive attitude the problems become smaller (right).
As a result you grow in stature, confidence and influence.*

In fact, both of the inner circles are both the same size.

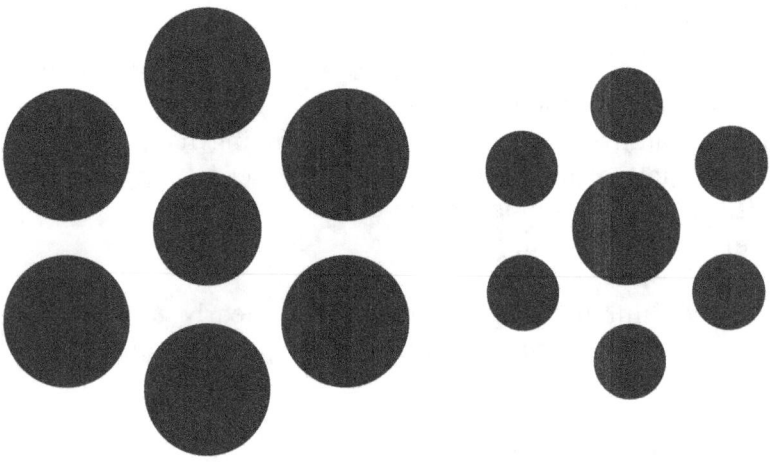

THE THREE P'S

The first 'P' is to make all of your affirmations
positive. The unconscious finds it easier to take in a message
couched in a positive way. So, if you want to create an
affirmation to stop eating foods that encourage you to put on
weight you would not say *"I do not eat chocolate"* or *"I will not*

eat chocolate" this will not be recognised by your unconscious. You would need to say "*I only eat healthy foods*".

Don't use 'get out' phrases like "*I'll try*" or "*I wish*" as both are a powerful admission of future failure. Whenever you use "*I'll try*" what you are really saying is that "*I will try, but I know that I will fail.*" You are admitting failure in advance.

You will have already experienced this yourself, how often has someone told you that they will try to change bad habits, try to stop smoking, try to eat less or try to be on time. Let me ask you, how often have they succeeded? - never, it doesn't happen. "*I'll try*" always means "*I will not, and I'm telling you this in advance*" so, never, never use this phrase in an affirmation.

As an aside, knowing the real meaning of the phrase "*I'll try*", is really useful when you are in negotiation with other people. They will often use "*I'll try*" when they expect not to deliver what you are asking for. Never let them get away with this, always insist on a definite yes or no in response to your questions - you are much more likely not to be disappointed!

Avoid using "*I wish*", this implies that you are not in control. If you are not in control then you can't be held responsible for any future failure. Then there is no incentive to succeed, because you have not committed yourself to the task - this in itself is enough to cause you to fail. Wish for things that are beyond your control, like winning the lottery, or the football pools - don't ever wish to lose weight.

You and you alone are responsible for your own actions - you and you alone can change the situation you are in. If you accept that you are responsible for your life, you will also accept that your destiny is created by you. This makes your life a physical manifestation of your thoughts, feelings and desires. Your destiny becomes what you think about. This is why you must take responsibility for your thoughts and your life - so don't wish or try, be positive, either decide to do something or not - and accept the consequences of your actions.

When you decide to use an affirmation always make it positive and totally focused on your goal.

The second 'P' for creating affirmations is to make them personal.

Always use the word I - by making them personal you attach an emotional trigger to the affirmation. This drives it deeper into the subconscious. Emotional triggers are known to have a greater effect on the subconscious - this helps to attach a chemical trigger to the affirmation, making it a more powerful, vivid instruction. This also makes it much easier to visualise the results of you positive affirmations - a technique that we will cover later.

The third 'P' is to make all of your affirmations present tense.

This might sound strange, and takes a little getting used to, but construct your affirmations as if they are already true, as if they already exist. Remember that the subconscious operates 'in the now', this is the only tense it understands.

If you remember the scary movie example used earlier, it clearly demonstrates how your subconscious reacts faithfully to the information you give it. Because even before the movie you would have known that at some point you would be scared by it - yet this knowledge did not stop your intense reaction. This third 'P' works in exactly the same way.

Afterwards thinking about that scary point in the movie would not have produced a physical reaction, the only time you tensed up, your heart started pounding and the adrenaline started pumping was when it happened. In the present, 'in the now'.

That is why all affirmations should be in the present tense as if they exist right now, don't use *"In 12 months time I will have lost 24lbs in weight"*, use *"I lose 1oz a day in weight"* or *"I weigh (your goal weight)"*.

By using these simple rules you can create your own powerful and personal affirmations that will help you change your self-concept.

Creating your own positive affirmations speeds up the re-programming process. Because they are more personal they will mean much more to you and will have a much greater effect in a shorter time span.

The following positive affirmations are the ones that have been used by people who are successful at weight loss.

"I act like a slim, trim person".
"I feel like a slim, trim person".

"I eat like a slim, trim person".
"I look like a slim, trim person".
"I behave like a slim, trim person".
"I think like a slim, trim person".

Although these can be used to great effect separately, they are more effective if used together and rounded off with:

"Because I am a slim, trim person".

I still use these on a regular basis. They just pop into my head, usually when I'm feeling good about myself. I also use them more when I need a bit of mental support, usually after a little over indulgence the night before.

THE NINETY DAY MENTAL DIET

Continually repeat your positive affirmations. Repeat them when you are in the bath, walking to the shops, in the car or at home. Repeat them all of the time because the more you repeat them the faster and further you drive them into your subconscious mind. Remember, repitition is the mother of skill. Repeat, repeat, repeat.

When we have a new thought, when we have an affirmation that alters our self image, that thought physically creates a new neural pathway in our brain. Continual repetition of that thought makes that pathway stronger and stronger, until it becomes dominant, and it is then that it becomes established as a habit pattern. That new thought or affirmation then replaces the old one to become a new part of our self-image.

It psychological studies have shown that it takes up to ninety days for a new habit pattern to be firmly established using positive affirmation. Dr C. Norman Shealy, founder of the American Holistic Medical Association believes that;

> *"Three months is a minimal time in which to develop a habit."*

After which you will start to think naturally about eating the right foods, because you will have changed your self-concept in that area.

Then you should continue to use affirmations to 'top-up' your new self-concept. This is important because previous habit patterns can take a long time to permanently suppress, especially when you are feeling low, or imbalanced.

A good metaphor is to think of bad habit patterns as weeds in a garden. Weeds will grow with no help at all, they will grow naturally and without effort. If you don't want your mind to be full of weeds, you will need to tend your mind on a regular basis.

Go on a ninety day 'mental diet' of using positive affirmations, and you'll soon notice the difference in your self-concept. You will soon notice the physical effects of the change in your self-concept - you will start to feel much better in yourself, and, of course, you will begin the process of losing weight.

I'm in control

This section deals with four key areas that you ought to look at to change your self-concept for the better. Although only indirectly linked to weight loss, these four cornerstone areas are vitally important to your development as a confident, happy and assured person. This has a major effect on your ability to lose and maintain weight loss. It's important that you address them before moving on to the lessons covering goal setting and visualisation.

These four cornerstones are increasing motivation, accepting responsibility, overcoming stress and banishing guilt. When you have mastered and are in control of these key areas, you will provide yourself the perfect mental foundation for the task ahead. The techniques you will learn here will help you to overcome many of life's little problems, long after you have reached your ideal weight and forgotten all about this old programme.

THE DESIRE WITHIN

To lose weight you need the right motivation. The motivation for all change in your life is desire. It is a selfish thing, you can only have the desire to change for yourself. If you had no desire to lose weight you would not even be studying this programme. The very fact that you are means that you have, and this programme will help you focus that desire and turn it outward in the form of taking action.

All desire to change must come from within, it is an intensely personal thing and one that is very simple to instil.

I would like to share with you the experience of a friend of mine called Martin. His experience contains a valuable lession in how to find the right motivation to give up a bad habit.

Two years ago Martin, who was a 40-a-day smoker, was at home watching television with his wife Jane and two young daughters, Sally and Gwen. When the sitcom that they were watching ended, a documentary on the dangers of smoking came on. Martin decided he really did not need to watch this and retired to the kitchen for a cigarette (because of the dangers of passive smoking, he never used to smoke in the lounge).

About fifteen minutes later his six year old daughter Sally burst into the kitchen crying hysterically. Assuming she had been fighting with her older sister, which was a fairly common occurrance, Martin scooped her up into his arms and tried to console her. Eventually she calmed down enough to sob out why she was so upset.

"Oh daddy, daddy please don't die!". She sobbed and flung her arms around her father.

Martin was shocked. *"I'm not going to die, little one."*

"They are killing you, they are killing you, and I love you so much. I don't want you to die." She was pointing accusingly toward the cigarette buring in the ash tray.

Martin quickly stubbed it out. *"There darling, it's gone. It's out now."*

Still she continued to cry *"I don't want you to leave me, I love you too much. Please, please don't die daddy, I want you to stay with me."*

Martin was gutted. He had always been able to justify his habit to himself, but to see the effect that his smoking was having on his little girl was devastating. He could not bear to see her in so much pain. He picked up the packet of cigarettes by the ash tray and crushed them, and threw them into the bin. He then turned to Sally and promised her that he would never smoke again. To this day he never has.

The pain of seeing the effect his smoking had on his daughter outweighed the pleasure that he gained from the habit. This was all the leverage he needed to stop smoking.

If you can find the right leverage you to can instantly change the bad habits of a lifetime.

This technique is well documented in psychology. The foundation of Dr Seigmund Freud's pain/pleasure principle is that we try to move away from pain and towards pleasure. Freud went on to suggest that all human behaviour is governed by this principle. So to move away from something you do not want (being overweight) you need to associate it with some form of pain. This pain can be emotional or physical.

This principle can be a difficult thing to practice because we instinctively avoid pain, but if you can bear with me for the next exercise, I guarantee that you will find it much easier to lose weight. For five minutes of pain (emotional) you will receive a lifetime's pleasure (successful weight loss). You will also gain a technique that you can use to change other bad habits you might have.

If you think back on any action you have taken, you will be able to remember a desire for change that caused it. For example, Martin originally started smoking to fit in with his 'peer group' at school - this need for social acceptance was stronger than the short term discomfort or the long term damage that smoking caused to his body. For Martin smoking was justified because it gave him more pleasure than pain, that was until he was made to review his priorities and change his behaviour.

The reason we take action is always to improve our situation, to be better off after the action than we were before it, to move away from pain and towards pleasure.

None of us will deliberately take a decision which we know will make us worse off than before. Without this desire for positive change there is no incentive and therefore no reason to change. So before committing yourself to losing weight, you need to measure your desire for change. For this exercise you will need a pen and a blank piece of A4 paper.

To measure your 'desire level' to do this ask yourself this one question. On a scale of 1 to 100, how much do I desire to lose weight?

Make a note of your score. Write it down.

Whatever your score or 'desire level', you can increase your motivation to change by using this simple exercise. It's guaranteed to increase your desire for change, if you follow the steps faithfully it works 100% of the time. There are no exceptions.

Write down a fact about being overweight (in the first person), then think of a possible outcome or consequence of this fact. Write down as many facts and possible consequences that you can think of . Try to make the facts bald and impersonal, then make the consequences specific, dramatic but possible. Below are three examples to set the style;

1. *Every stone I'm overweight I take 12 years off my life - If I die young I would miss my only daughters' wedding.*

2. *Being overweight makes me breathless - soon I will not have the energy to walk up a flight of stairs.*

3. *I find it embarrassing to wear a swimsuit - I look like a stranded whale on the beach. I think people laugh at me behind my back.*

Stop reading for a moment. Now think of or if possible write out as many facts and consequences as you can think of and please take your time. You should be able to think of between 20 and 30. Some people having done this exercise have come up with over 60!

Look at your sheet of paper, look at the consequences of the situation you are in. Remember all of them are possible outcomes unless you decide to take action.

Then ask yourself again on a scale of 1 to 100, how much do you desire to lose weight?

Now, of the facts and consequences you have in front of you pick three which have the most dramatic consequences. Circle them, and taking each in turn read (out loud) the consequence. Close your eyes and spend between thirty seconds to one minute trying to imagine the consequence of your actions. Try to picture how this will effect your life and the lives of the people you care for.

Now imagine what it would be like in five years time if you allow this to continue unchanged. How would it affect you? How would it affect your family? How would it affect you work?

Now picture a food that makes you fat. One that you know you must eat less of to stop this consequence becoming a reality. Associate the pleasure you get from eating this food with the consequence, and the emotions you have just been feeling. Imagine every bite of that food is pushing you closer to that consequence - every bite turning that consequence into reality. Now while this is still vivid in your mind ask yourself:

On a scale of 1 to 100, how much do you want to lose weight?

Repeat this exercise for all three consequences.

Now, on a scale of 1 to 100, how much do you want to lose weight?

If you complete this exercise two things will have happened, your desire to lose weight will have increased. If it was already high, you have reinforced your desire with some very powerful motivations.

You will certainly have less desire to eat those three foods, which in itself will help you lose weight dramatically!

Now you have the desire not to eat those foods, you need to anchor it with immediate positive action. If you have any of those foods in the house throw them in the bin.

If you are not in a position to bin them, imagine a situation when you will next encounter them. Imagine throwing the food against a wall, whilst screaming "No Fat! No, Fat!!". Picture the surprised looks on the faces of the people around you.

If, of course, having thrown the food in the bin or against the wall, you find yourself weakening, just remember before you eat that food the consequence your actions will have. How this small thing will have a big effect on your health in the future. If you then still choose to eat it, it's your decision, you know the consequences and you are totally responsible for your own life.

Whatever it's outcome.

TAKING RESPONSIBILITY FOR YOUR LIFE

Accepting responsibility is one of the chief traits of the well balanced, mature human being. By taking responsibility for your life you gain one very important thing. Control. The more responsibility you accept for your life the more control you have.

It also means one other very important thing, that from the moment you accept responsibility for your life there are no more excuses.

Ultimately, we must recognise that we are responsible for our attitude and behaviour. Now you need to seize control of that responsibility and use it in a more focused, constructive and positive way.

To do this you need to take control of situations that have caused you frustration, resentment or anger in the past. If in the past a particular situation that has caused you to feel a negative emotion, try the technique below to ragain control of your feelings.

If you have ever harboured resentment about a situation, this will play on your mind. You will remember the injustice. You will feel the hurt. Whenever you remember that situation all of the negative feelings associated with it will come flooding back.

Do these feelings make you feel good about yourself? No they do not - in fact, just the reverse. Every time you think this way what you are really doing is allowing that person who hurt you to control your emotions. You are giving them control of your thoughts, and are responsible for giving them this power over you. Do they deserve to have this control over your emotions? I think not.

Try this exercise in accepting responsibility for your actions.

Think back to a situation when someone else has hurt you. Perhaps a spiteful comment from someone you thought of as good friend, or being publicly humilliated at work by a superior or even being taken advantage of by a stranger. Take a minute to think of a specific situation. Remember it as if it were happening right now, and ask yourself these questions.

Do you still harbour resentment for this person? How long has this negative emotion been eating away at you? Do you still blame them for the situation? When you think about the situation does your stomach knot up? Does your feeling of injustice increase?

I'm sure you can answer yes to one or more of these feelings. Now, be honest with yourself and analyse the circumstance around that situation. Look at the situation from the other persons point of view;

What was their motivation? What was it about your actions that made them react the way they did? In hindsight, could you have found a comprimse?

Now look at the situation from a third party point of view;

What would their view of the situation have been? How would a third party have apportioned responsibility for the dispute?

Having considered these two points of view were you not also partially responsible for the situation? If you consider any situation from these other points of view, you will realise that in most instances, you contributed to the dispute. You were partly responsible.

If you want to be totally free of feelings of injustice, anger, frustration and lack of control, you need to accept responsibility for your actions.

This is an easy thing to do, while thinking about the situation, repeat the following affirmation;

"I am responsible."

You will probably say it angrily through gritted teeth, but say it again:

"I am responsible."

and again

"I am responsible."

And again, and again, and again.

"I am responsible, I am responsible, I am responsible."

It gets easier doesn't it? It reduces the amount of negative feeling associated with the situation, and allows you to put it aside.

Now, that the situation is no longer important, why not forgive the other person for their actions? You don't have to do it publicly, or like them afterwards. We have all done silly, stupid and senseless things and sometimes we do them to other people. Find the compassion in your heart to forgive them.

If you can do this you will totally and completely free you from the negative feelings associated with the situation. If you can do this you will put the situation behind you forever. You will have regained control over your thoughts, try it, you will feel a lot better afterwards.

FREE YOURSELF FROM STRESS

Over 90% of the population worry about aspects of their lives. When people worry on a regular basis they develop into a state of stress. Stress has an outward and inward destructive effect on the body.

Outwardly many people try to relieve stress by overeating and drinking and we all know the consequences of those actions!

Inwardly stress releases adrenaline into the blood stream, this in turn produces a number of physical responses. Blood pressure rises. Muscles tense. Breathing becomes rapid and shallow.

If this continues for any length of time we show signs of premature aging. So much energy is being used on the physical effects of stress, that there is not enough for you body to effectively renew itself.

Stress is the great illness of this century. At any one time over 8% of the population are suffering from a stress related illness. Stress often manifestes itself as Migrane, Flu, Backache, Acne, Ashtma, Diabetes, Hypertension, Ulceration and many other common illnesses.

Stress is the body's physical reaction to worry and tension. It's effects can be devastating. Yet stress can be really easy to reduce or exclude from your life.

I know, because I'm an expert on the subject of stress. In my early twenties I was diagnosed with a stress related Peptic Ulcer. I thought I had a high pressure job, and worried about it so much that I made myself ill. Painfully ill. But, within six months I was totally cured and have had no problems since. I used no medication during this time, I just developed a strategy that would reduce my stress levels permanently. Now I find very few things make me worry and I rarely feel 'stressful' about anything.

I would like to share with you my strategy of reducing stress levels. It is simple and effective. If it worked for me it will work for you.

Stress is the body's reaction to prolonged worry. Worry is the fear of change or possibility of change in your current circumstances. Worry is always caused by indecision which leads to thinking about the various 'what if' scenarios. The more indicision the more variables there are and the more you worry. As soon as you make a decision to take action and follow a certain path you regain control of a situation, eliminate the variables and the worry disappears.

Let me show you the best method of making worry dissapear, it works 99.9% of the time. First, write down exactly what it is that you are worried about.

Second, write down the very worst thing that can happen as a consequence of that situation. When you see the worst case scenario written on paper most worries seem much less daunting. Hardly worth worrying about, in fact.

If the consequence still disturbes you, make a plan of action to avoid the worst case scenario. Write down what action you can take and how much time you have to take it. Then decide to take positive action based on your plan to change the possible outcome. Commit yourself to doing everything in your power to change the outcome.

The last thing you should do is resolve to accept the worst should it happen.

Taking this action puts you back in control of the situation and eliminates any worry caused by indecision. It also makes you face the worst outcome, and gives you a plan to improve upon it.

When I first used this strategy to cure my work related ulcer I wrote:

I worry that my boss thinks I'm incompetent.

The worst case scenario is that I will lose my job.

My plan of action is to ask my boss exactly how I can improve my skills, and be more valuable to the company. I will do this tomorrow.

If the worst happens I can always find another job.

Those fifty seven words stopped me worrying about my job, reduced my stress level and cured my Peptic Ulcer. In fact my boss was so impressed with the interest I had shown, he arranged additional training for me. He also told me that he had never doubted my competance, so I had been worrying over nothing all along.

Spend five minutes writing down the reasons that you worry. Once you have used this strategy I'm sure that many of them will simply disappear and for the rest you will have a plan to eliminate them.

FREE YOURSELF FROM GUILT

The last of the four cornerstones we need to look at is guilt. We have all felt guilty in our lives. We have all tried to make others feel guilty.

Guilt is an emotion that you were taught at an early age. It is an emotion that is passed on from generation to generation, you were probably taught it by your mother or father. The reason that we are all taught it, is that it is such an effective method of controlling our behaviour.

If you are aware of how people who use guilt to manipulate you and have the strategies to avoid being manipulated, you can retain control of your actions. Remember we, are happy to the degree that we feel in control of a situation.

There are two types of people who use guilt as a control device, they are:

Guilt catchers - These are the people who seem happy to jump up and take responsibility for a problem - even if it was not their fault. They then use the situation that they find themselves in to metaphorically beat themselves. It seems that they just love to heap blame upon themselves. They just love to be guilty of something. Guilt catchers are willing victims of the other type of guilt users. The Guilt throwers.

Guilt throwers - These are the people you have to watch out for and have the strategies to deal with. Guilt throwers are the people who are constantly reminding you of you responsibilities, obligations and endebtedness to others. These people like to manipulate you by making you feel guilty. The strange thing is that they probably do not even realise that they are doing it, for it has become such a natural part of their character.

Fortunately there is an easy way deal with these guilt throwers. Whenever you are in a situation where you become aware that the other person is trying to use guilt as a method of control, simply stop the conversation. Look them in the eye, smile and say "*You're not trying to make me feel guilty are you?*" They will immediately reply "*No, of course not."* and the conversation can then continue.

But be warned they will try to use guilt again in the conversation, usually within one or two minutes. When it happens again (and it will) simply go through the process of stopping the conversation again, smiling and asking the question. Do this every time they try to use guilt on you. Sooner or later they will realise that this particular method of control will not work and they will stop.

If you use this strategy to deal with guilt throwers they will never be able to make you feel guilty again.

Now that you have the techniques to increase your motivation, have taken responsibility for your own life, have the means to banish stress from your life and have freed yourself from guilt you are now ready to tackle the next key step to effective weight loss.

The importance of goal setting

In an interview to determine what made people successful, Bunker Hunt who went from a bankrupt cotton farmer to a self-made billionare in just 20 years, was asked the great secret of his success. He thought about this question carefully and then replied "*You know, there are only two things you really need to achieve success. Before I undertake any venture I always ask myself these two things.*

First I clearly define exactly what it is that I want from the venture. Then I estimate exactly what this would cost in personal and financial terms. If I still consider the venture worthwhile, I resolve to pay that price."

That's it. It's that easy. This two step philosophy took Bunker Hunt from rags to one of the richest men in the world in just 30 years. He started hundreds of successful companies. He made millions of dollars for himself and others - and now you know the secret of his success.

If you have a clearly defined goal, understand the cost and decide to pay the price you have given yourself the focus to achieve that goal.

Bunker Hunt went on to say that, in his opinion, where the majority of people fail is clearly defining exactly what it is that they want. The rest of this chapter gives you practical techniques that will help you focus on what exactly it is that you want and the methodology to drive your goals deep into your subconscious and keep them there.

Losing weight is just as simple, all you have to do is set yourself a goal weight and eat less until you reach that goal weight. Medical opinion, weight loss and health experts are in total agreement on this point. To lose weight you must consume less energy than your body uses. For the average woman that's under 1,900 calories per day and for men less than 2,400 - there are no short cuts. As yet there are no magic tablets or miracle solutions. Or put another way, being overweight is simply your body's way of telling you that you eat more than you need!

Goals, like affirmations, programme your unconscious mind at a deep level. The big difference between affirmations and goals is that goals define the target that you are aiming at, whereas affirmations help you develop the mind set to hit that target.

Knowing what you are aiming at allows you to focus on the right strategies to get exactly what you want. If you are not already getting what you want, could it be that you have not exactly defined what you want and how to get it?

There is dramatic evidence from America that suggests that habitual goal setting is the key difference between over and under achievement.

A study conducted at Harvard University asked graduating seniors if they had clearly focused, written goals defining their career and financial development. Only 3% said that they had. Twenty years later the graduating seniors were contacted again, and it was found that the 3% who had made clear goals were at the top of their chosen professions and were worth more in net terms than the other 97% combined.

The study also measured other possible contributory factors such as racial origin, intelligence, status, sex and education, none of which were shown to make a difference. The only common denominator between the financially successful and the rest was their ability to focus on and define their goals. This finding has been replicated in a number of different studies in the USA. The results are always the same.

Based on this type of evidence, I suggest that we study goal setting in more detail. You might not want to use goal setting to become fabulously wealthy, and that's ok. The goal setting techniques that I will share with you are equally effective for losing weight!

A goal is defined in The Oxford English Dictionary as *"the object of effort or ambition, the destination of a journey."*

The reason that goals are so effective is that they provide a focus for our efforts. By using goals to channel our energies we are much more efficient, more purposeful and as a consequence, more successful.

We as individuals need to be very focused on what we want for two reasons.

Firstly, life is too short, and your resources to limited too be wasting them on ill defined vague objectives. You may have heard the now popular phrase "Don't work harder, work smarter" this perfectly sums up the way we can rapidly achieve our objectives.

Secondly, we live in a world where the only sure thing is change. Unexpected change makes us feel insecure, yet none of us fear change for the better. In this world of change goals provide the necessary focus for positive change. Without properly constructed, clearly defined goals you have little or no control over the direction of your life. As Brian Tracy, an American self-development guru once said *"If your are travelling nowhere any road will take you there."* Goals help you shape the way that you change.

GOAL SETTING IS VITAL TO WEIGHT LOSS

Well defined goals will help you to shape the change in your life, and are extremely useful as part of your weight loss strategy. They help you define exactly what it is that you want to achieve.

To be effective, goals need to be specific and measurable - if it is vague or indistinct it is not a goal, it is just a hope or a wish. If you remember from chapter three, a wish is just an admission of failure in advance.

You will already have had some personal experience of this. You will have yourself, or know somebody who has, said *"I really need to lose some weight.",* or *"I really hope this diet works."* or *"I'm trying to lose weight."* or even *"I must lose weight."*

Let me ask you, have these people lost weight? Are they still saying the same things? Do you actually believe they are ever going to lose weight?

No. Yes. No. They are probably no further forward than when they started. They may well be working hard, but they are not working smart. To work smart they have to have clearly defined what it is they want.

SMALL DECISIONS SHAPE OUR LIVES

If you have ever started a new weight loss programme, you have almost certainly decided to restrict the food in your diet. You will have been enthusiastic, positive and keen to cut out the foods that make you put weight on.

But, if you are typical of the 98% of us that have failed to maintain a weight loss programme, you will have drifted back to those very foods that you had vowed to give up only hours, days or weeks before.

Psychologically there is a simple explanation for this behaviour. The desire to lose weight was not as strong as the desire for those fattening foods. This is a very common, natural and well documented phenomenon.

Think back to a particular situation where this has happened to you. Think back to the exact time when you broke your diet. As you reached for the chocolate cake, the glass of wine, the bag of chips, remember what you were thinking.

You didn't care about losing weight, at that exact moment in time all that mattered was to satisfy your immediate craving. While you were eating you felt great, satisfied and happy. Only afterwards would you have felt guilty, ashamed, dissapointed, but by then it was too late.

The habit pattern that determined your desire for that fattening food was much stronger than the new 'diet' habit pattern that you were trying to form.

When you use the positive affirmation, goal setting and visualisation techniques described, you will dramatically increase your chances of successfully losing weight. But there is one additional technique you can use that will virtually guarantee your success. It's logic is so obvious, so fundamental, so simple and so personal, you will be amazed that you have not read about it before.

Before I explain it, I would like to ask you a question. Can you think back to a time in your life when a small thing that you did made a dramatic impact on future events?

Perhaps you decided to go to a social event, at which you met your partner. Or perhaps you decided to apply for a job, which subsequently shaped your career.

Take a moment to think back to a small decision or action you have taken, that has in the long term shaped your life.

If you look back on your life, you will realise that it has been shaped by all of the small decisions that you have made. Life is made up of small decisions, that dramatically affect our lives.

LOSE JUST ONE OUNCE A DAY

Traditional weight loss programmes ask you to dramatically change your eating habits. They ask you to give up many of the foods you enjoy. This, as we have all experienced, causes conflict with your established habit patterns. This causes cravings for these exact foods, which in turn cause you to weaken and eventually fail.

I ask you to consider an alternative.

Consider not dieting. Consider not restricting the foods that you eat. Just consider losing such a small amount of weight every day, an amount so tiny that you knew you could not possibly fail. Consider losing just one ounce a day.

Imagine how easy it would be to lose such a small amount each day. If you lost just one ounce per day in weight, you would lose about 2lb a month or around 2 stone in one year.

Would you like to lose two stone in weight over a period of a year without restricting the foods that you eat?

If you answered yes, I've got some great news for you. You can!

To do this you do not have to dramatically change your existing eating style. To lose one ounce a day all you would need to do is eat between 230 and 260 calories less per day. This technique reminds me of a saying that I heard many years ago and that has always stuck with me: *"Inch by inch, life's a cinch, yard by yard life's hard"*

There are two tried and tested methods that you can use to achieve the goal of losing one ounce a day.

The first method is to decide on something specific that you eat and cut it out of your diet. For example: it could be one less chocolate bar, two bags of crisps, half a bag of salted peanuts or perhaps one large glass of red wine less a day. It dosen't even have to be the same thing everyday, you can vary the food cut out dependant on your own preferences. If you examine your eating patterns throughout the day, you will find that there are many opportunities to lose something so small from your diet. If this is still hard try substituting a healthier food in the place of the one that you have chosen to cut out.

The other method is to leave 10% of your meals on the plate untouched. This takes slightly more willpower than the first method but is highly effective. Alternatively you could prepare 10% less in the first place - this would also produce the desired result.

Whichever method you decide to use you have to be committed to follow it for at least two weeks. This is important because by then this change will have become a habit - and you will probably be looking at other areas where you can change your diet for the better.

Using either of these two methods is guaranteed to help you lose two stone in twelve months. If losing just two stone in a year seems a small amount, I'd like to ask you exactly how much weight did you lost last year using your existing methods?

The reason that this strategy is so effective is that your existing eating habits are only subtly altered. But, the really neat effect of this strategy is that you have to analyse your own existing food intake and modify it in a way that perfectly suits you.

So, why don't you try it?

Think of your diet and decide right now, what little change you could make, that will make a massive difference to your weight, over the next twelve months. It need not be the same change every day, or even the same method, just as long as you take positive action. When you do take action think to yourself "that's my ounce for today" and feel good about yourself. Think of the difference that little change will have in just twelve months time.

That's it. That's all you need to do to lose weight. No diets, no pain, no hunger, no cravings and no exercise. Just resolve to make one tiny change in your eating habits, and that change will dramatically improve your life.

Could you do that? Could you change just one tiny eating habit if it guaranteed to help you lose two stone in weight? I think you could, and the best thing of all is it's your choice. You are in total control, after all you know that you are totally responsible for the way you look and feel.

Decide right now which method you will use, and resolve to make that little change.

An interesting thing about the 'losing one ounce a day' technique is that it immediately changes your attitude to weight loss.

DO THE LINES BULGE IN THE CENTRE?

No they do not, it is only the radiating lines that make them appear to do so. Don't let outside influences interfere with your direction. Keep your goals stright and true and you will reach your desired destination.

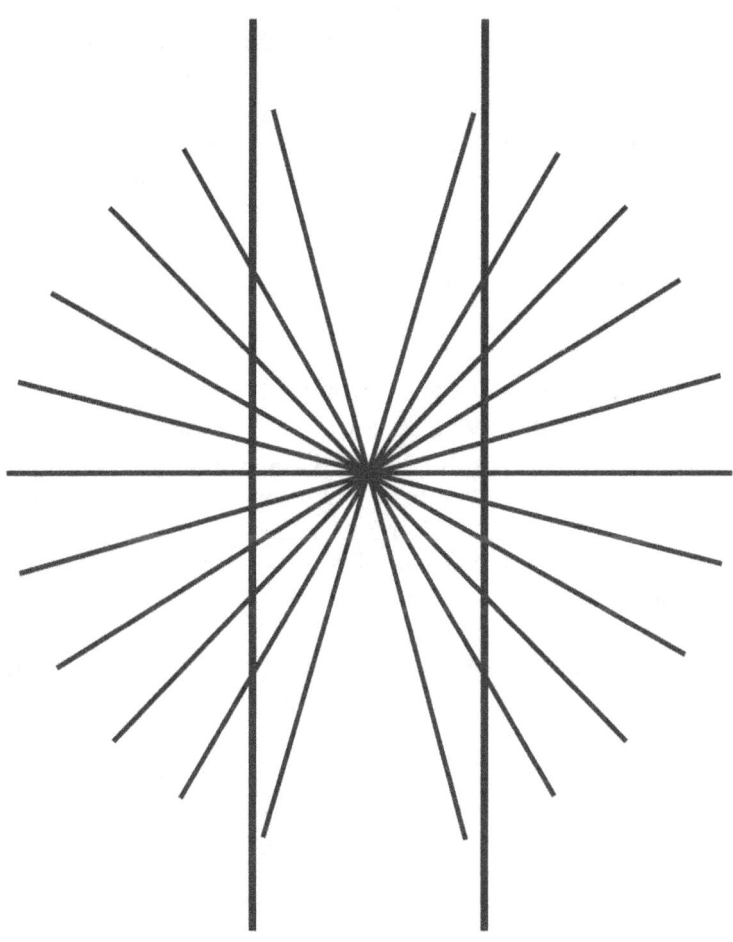

Because what you give up is so small, it's so much easier for your desire to lose weight to overcome the desire of your existing eating habit patterns. Even if you do weaken and eat something you had planned to avoid simply substitute something else in its place.

I have taught this strategy to many people, and it works. Don't be put off because it does not appear to give a quick fix or an instant dramatic change in your weight. That is the strategies great strength.

When I initially developed this strategy, I found that I was cutting out a number of little things. At first I stopped visiting the office tuck box for chocolate in the afternoon. Then I stopped eating pastries with my lunch and substituted fruit. Next, I cut milk from my tea and substituted lemon.

The process has not stopped since those first small changes. I immediately noticed the difference, I felt healthier, I felt more in control. Then when I started to lose weight, the motivation for change was dramatically increased. I actually lost the two stone in just six months. Many others who have used this technique have had similar experiences.

Paul Butler wrote to me nine months after using this strategy:

"I'm amazed, I'm healthy, I'm three stone lighter. Even now I look back at the person I was and cannot believe the vast difference such small changes have made. The lose an ounce a day method was a marvellous piece of advice. Thank you."

No diet, dieter Dawn Porter observed:

"You were wrong about losing two stone in a year, I did it in eight months! So, far I've lost over four stone. People ask me what the secret is...it's losing one ounce a day, every day."

Four months into her 'no diet' Danielle Rocca joked:

"I laughed when you suggested I lose one ounce a day, but when I started to lose weight..."

If you resolve to lose just one ounce a day, you will achieve similar results. In a year's time, usually less, you will have lost two stone in weight - without restricting the foods you eat or substantially changing your diet. It really is that simple as long as your goal is to "Lose one ounce a day, two pounds a month, two stone per year."

Remember that it really is the small decisions that you make that dramatically change your life. Go on, make a small decision, dramatically change your life. Do it now.

The 'lose an ounce a day' is simply a weight loss strategy defined as a goal. You can set your own goals, for any part of your life. I have sifted through numerous books on goal setting and have compiled what I believe to be the very best techniques available; If you use them you will achieve things in months that would normally taken you years. You will amaze yourself at how quickly you can develop and improve all aspects of your life.

Ideally you should start with four or five goals that you want to achieve within a year. They should cover your personal life, your career and your personal development. When you write down your goals use the six rules below - they are distilled from the very best teaching on the subject.

WRITE YOUR GOALS DOWN

You must write you goals down on paper. Until they are committed to paper they are not really goals at all - they are just hopes and wishes. The act of writing your goals down turns them from thoughts into something real and tangible. Writing goals down gives them substance.

Write exactly what it is that you want to achieve. Describe it in minute detail, the more accurate you are the more focused the goal is. At the same time write down the benefits of achieving the goal. Write down as many benefits as you can imagine. If you have one good reason for achieving a goal you will be slightly motivated, if you have one hundred you will become unstoppable.

Revise your list of goals on a regular basis. Update them and don't be afraid to modify them to suit new circumstances.

MAKE YOUR GOALS BELIEVABLE

To set a goal of losing eight stone in a year is very commendable - but probably not very realistic if you have failed in the past. All of your goals should be achievable otherwise your subconscious will not accept them. If your subconscious doesn't accept a goal as believable it will not start to act on it, and you will fail. In this instance a goal of losing two stone per year is more believable, and therefore likely to succeed.

Your goals should have about a 50/50 chance of becoming reality. A goal that has a 100% chance of success is not a goal at all, just an activity. A goal with a 50% chance of success will force you to stretch yourself in order to achieve it.

MAKE YOUR GOALS ACHIEVABLE

If you have a large goal, it can often seem daunting. This can make it appear to be harder to achieve than it really is. For example, to lose two stone in weight might seem impossible, until you break it down to two pounds a month and then to one ounce a day.

One ounce a day seems such a small amount that the goal appears to be much easier. Break down your goals into small bite sized chunks - your chances of success will be increased dramatically.

GIVE YOUR GOAL A STRICT TIME LIMIT

Set yourself a time limit for your goals. Decide on a deadline by which you will have succeeded or failed to achieve your goal. This helps to focus the mind on the task in hand. Making goals measurable helps your to gauge how close you are to them and what you have to do to make them happen. A benefit of making goals measurable is that, if you are ahead of your target, this is a great boost to your confidence and self-esteem.

ACT AS IF THE GOAL HAS ALREADY BEEN ACHIEVED

Think of your goals as already having been achieved. If you have a goal to lose two stone in weight adopt the mind set of the new lighter you, pretend that it has already happened. Act in a manner consistant with how you would be if you were two stone lighter. Goals are just a means of focussing the subconscious and remember from chapter two that the subconscious only operates 'in the now'.

In this way goal setting works exactly like the third 'P' for affirmations - act as if your desired outcome has already happened.

KEEP YOUR GOALS PRIVATE

Having taken all of the steps outlined above, there is one last and very important thing you need to do in order to succeed. That is to keep your goals to yourself.

A number of studies have show that if you tell your peer group about your plans, hopes and dreams the typical reactions to them are negative. People who do not use goals to direct their lives will react by telling you that *"you should not have ideas above your station."* or that *"You don't have the ability to succeed"* or even *"you are asking for too much, you will fail."*

This type of negative reaction from your peer group is enough to make you fail at your chosen task. Every study has shown that the reaction of your peer group is a key determinant to your success or failure.

There is one exception to this rule - share your goals with anyone who is going to be positive, encouraging or who can help you achieve them.

The first time I used goal setting I wrote down ten goals that I wanted to achieve in one year. These goals covered my personal life, my working career, my personal development. One of them was to develop and publish this programme. Within eight months I had achieved nine of my original goals, you are reading the tenth. During that time I also achieved an additional six goals. The combination of these achievements has had a dramatic and positive impact on my life.

The results achieved by using these goal setting techniques are by no means unusual, many people who focus on specific goals achieve far more dramatic results. I have a friend who increased his salary from £25,000 per year to £250,000 a year in just twelve months using these goal setting techniques. Another friend went from being a secretary in a dead end job to becoming the chief executive of a multi-national company just four years later.

There is no doubt that goal setting can help you achieve the things that you want from life far more quickly than any other method. You really should try goal setting, it will change your life. And your weight.

The power of Visualisation

Visualisation is simply a technique that we all use to communicate with our subconscious. When we think about what we experience, we create it in our heads. This process is called visualisation.

All of us represent things that are important to us in our minds, all of the time. It's how your memory works. It's why you can 'hear' the bars of your favourite tune. It's how you can see the face of a loved one. Visualisation is a normal, natural function of your mind.

If you consciously attempt to develop this natural skill it can increase ability to perform certain tasks. For example, all top athletes visualise their desired outcome from competition. By seeing themselves performing sucessfully, they 'programme' their bodies to act in a manner consistant with that success.

We can use it to condition ourselves in exactly the same way. Can you remember a time when you were feeling stressed out? Most of us feel stressful, anxious or pent-up at some time, but you can reduce the effect of stress using visualisation.

What is your stress level this precise moment? Think of a number between 0 and 100. Zero being totally relaxed, one hundred being totally stressed out. How stressed are you, right now? Pick a number.

Read the following passage, then re-run it in your head. When you re-run the passage either close your eyes or focus on the image below.

TAKE A WALK ON A SUN DRENCHED BEACH

Now, take a moment to think about walking along a sun-drenched, deserted sandy beach.

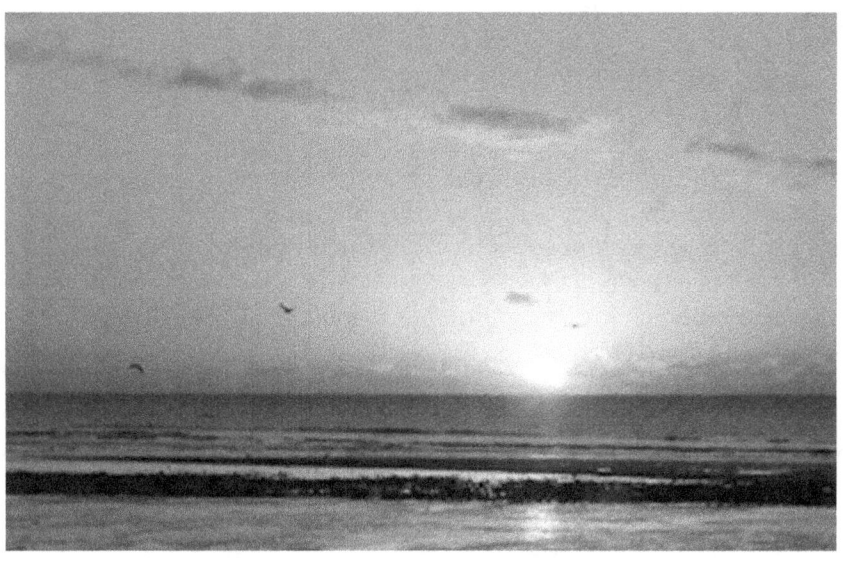

You are walking barefoot in the sand, you can feel the pleasantly warm sand under you feet. To your left magnificent palm trees tower overhead. On your right is the vast expanse of ocean.

Looking out to sea you marvel at the constantly changing colour of the sea. Surf is rolling onto the beach, you can hear the sounds of the crashing waves and taste the salt spray on your lips. The sun is high in the sky, you feel it's warmth on your head and shoulders, despite the cooling onshore breeze.

You reach down and pick up a beautiful shell half hidden in the sand and run your fingers over it's rough contours. Wandering on you remember that lunch will soon be served back at your beachhut, you can already taste the tropical fruits that await you...

On a scale of 0 to 100, how relaxed do you feel right now?

To make any sense of the passage, above you would have needed access to similar memories that you have already experienced. Or constructed them from other similar experiences, or even drawn on reference from remembered t.v. programmes, books or films. You were visualising the scene.

The interesting thing is that you would have been using the same neurological pathways to represent the imagined experience as you would if you had actually been walking on the beach.

Your may have imagined the beach hut full of tropical fruits, but the expectation that the image triggered, was real enough.

The effects of what we think have a very real effect on the body. You probably experienced a difference while visualising the passage. Because of the subject matter, I was gambling on the fact that those memories evoked were pleasant ones. Because you can only think about one thing at a time, the pleasant memories, were replacing any stressful feelings that you might have been thinking. Thus reducing your 'stress level'.

Did it work, was your stress level lower after reading the passage? I have used this technique at seminars all over the country. and typically about 15% of people will have reduced their stress level by 10 to 30 points. 65% of people will have reduced their stress level by 5 to 10 points, and 20% of people experience little (1 to 5 points) or no change. I've never encounted anyone who has had their stress level increase!

For those who do not experience a difference, there is a more powerful variation on the technique. You can try this, exchange the beach scene for something that is personal to you. Remember a specific time when you felt happy, relaxed and totally at peace with yourself..

Where were you?

How did you feel?

What made that time so special?

Think on this for a few minutes. Then score your

'stress level' again.

Visualisation is a two way process and can be used to programme the sub conscious at a deep level. The technique requires no special skill or discipline, although like every skill you have mastered, the more you practice it the easier it becomes. Remember that repitition is the mother of skill.

We will use this technique to speed up your weight loss by focusing on your desired outcome. This will improve your will power, your desire to lose weight and to lead to subtle, positive improvements in your eating habits.

To try this technique, you should ideally find a quiet room where you will not be disturbed. In the room you will need a comfortable chair in which you can rest comfortably. A sound system on which you can play some melodic, instrumental background music, my personal favourite is Chariots of Fire by Vangelis. You will also need a pen and an A4 piece of blank paper.

Now, sit in that chair with your legs uncrossed, with your feet together and flat on the floor. You should have your arms by your side or folded in your lap, whichever feels the most comfortable.

Now close your eyes.

Take between three and six regular deep breaths to relax. When you breathe in, breathe from the abdomen, not the chest, as this enables you to fill the lungs properly and make more efficient use of the oxygen. Also breathe in for four seconds, hold the breath for four seconds, and exhale for four seconds. Maintaining a relaxed, comfortable rhythm is the desired outcome.

THE WEIGHT ESCALATOR

You are now ready to try a simple visualisation exercise called 'the weight escalator'. I developed this exercise in 1995, and have used it very sucessfully in seminars around the U.K. Many people find it gives them a unique insight into the small changes they need to make in their eating habits.*

*Authors Note. If you have it, this is the last exercise on the 'tip and techniques' audio, available from jimbrackin.com. If you would like to do it together, I recommend playing the tape at this point.

With your eyes still closed, picture yourself standing at the top of an escalator. Below, in a beautiful foyer, decorated in exotic pot plants and elegant seating, you can see an important social gathering. All of your closest friends and family are there. As you travel down the escalator you magically begin to shed all of your excess weight. By the time you reach the bottom you are at your ideal weight. You step off the escalator to join your friends. You are wearing clothes that show off this new, slim you.

See this picture of yourself at your ideal weight. The weight you would choose to be if nothing stood in your way. Then form a firm, clear image of yourself at this ideal weight. Try to hold this mental image, clearly in your mind and ask yourself the following questions:

How do you feel?
How do you look?
What sort of clothes are you wearing?
What types of food would you eat?
Do other people like you?
Do people find you more attractive?
Take a while to think on this image of the ideal you.

This image of the ideal you will make you feel good about yourself. It will make you feel happier, more confident, more self-assured. This is how you should, and could feel all of the time - it is your natural state.

Now while you are still in this relaxed state, go back to the question what types of food do you eat? Mentally list all of the foods you would need to eat to make the ideal weight you a reality.

Compare that list with your existing diet. Are there any foods you are eating now that the ideal you would not? Are there any foods that you are not eating now that the ideal you would?

By answering these questions your subconscious mind has given you clues on how to successfully lose weight. It has told you exactly the type of foods you need to eat, and how you need to feel in order to turn that ideal vision into reality. Now you need to take your own advice and resolve to adjust your diet. Start to consciously include the foods that will move you towards your perfect weight and eliminate or avoid all of those foods that hold you back. This might not be easy at first but, the very fact that you have the ability to picture the ideal you with imagination and emotion, means that you have it in your ability to make this vision a reality.

One method you can use to speed up this process is to make a list. Writing down your thoughts, aims and goals transforms them from ideas into a tangible reality. I suggest you draw two columns on your sheet of paper, one for column good foods, one for bad. List all of the foods you thought of in each category. Study this record and commit it to memory, and remember it when you are tempted by the wrong foods. After a few weeks repeat the exercise and revise your list.

The list will serve as an aide-memoire for the things you need to change in your diet. If you undertake this visualisation exercise in a few months time, you will be surprised at the change in the foods you list. That is assuming that you have acted on your own advice.

If you find taking action difficult or need some extra encouragement then the next visualisation exercise will help.

I call this the Core Reasons technique, because it enables you to understand the behaviour patterns that make you overweight - and the underlying reasons behind them. It also provides you with a proven method of changing that undesired behaviour pattern. This technique has been used all over the world to break thousands of people out of bad habits. It's previously been used to stop smoking, reduce the desire to drink and also to cure phobias. I have adapted it to be used specifically for weight loss.

THE CORE REASONS TECHNIQUE

For this exercise you need to find a quiet place where you will not be disturbed. Using the techniques described earlier ease yourself into a calm and relaxed state. You will need a pen and paper to hand for this technique.

In part one of the Core Reasons technique you will ask yourself a series of questions. The answers or situations will pop into your head. Consider these answers, then move on to the next question. It's important that you write your answers down. before you move on to the next question. Answer all of the questions in sequence honestly, accurately and with care - the more detailed your answers are, the more effective this technique will be. (In brackets I've given a ficticious set of answers, to show you how the technique works.)

———————

In part two you will visualise a series of positive outcomes based on your answers to the questions.

Question One. Identify exactly how you have become overweight.

(Example: As a child, my parents always rewarded me with sweets. I associated sweets with gaining approval. Now whenever I need to boost my spirits I have something sweet. This is the basis of many of my bad eating habits.)

Question Two. Exactly how and when does this happen?

(Example: I constantly pick at chocolate bars, buscuits and soft drinks. Usually during the day, especially an hour or two before a meal.)

Question Three. What drives you to take this action and keep repeating it?

(Example: I get urges for sweet things, I'm not really hungry but I can't resist them. I like chocolate bars with my afternoon coffee. Sometimes I have a craving for the chocolate, but most of the time it's just a habit)

Question Four. What positive intention have you really tried to achieve by using this type of behaviour?

(Example: I like to spoil myself, I like a little bit of indulgence. It's a need for comfort, the desire to have a good feeling, especially when I'm feeling low.)

Question Five. What has this behaviour cost you in terms of your weight?

(Example: I am three stone overweight, despite dieting on a regular basis. Despite my good intentions, I always break my diets by eating chocolate. I eat about one to two bars of chocolate a day - that's about 375 calories. In a year that adds up to 136,875 calories I don't really need. 136,800 calories equates to 45 lbs in weight* which is about what I'm overweight. It also cost me my self-esteem, I'm uncomfortable in the summer - especially on the beach. I can't get about as easily as I used to, I get short of breath very quickly.)   * Author's note. A pound of fat roughly equals 3,000 calories.

Question Six. Is there a way to achieve the same result without the negative side effects? Think of three alternatives.

(Example: Alternative one, I'll have something sweet that isn't chocolate. I really like dried apricots, I'll keep a bag to hand for mid afternoon coffee. Alternative two, When I start to feel low I will play my favourite piece of music to cheer myself up - before I get depressed enough to crave chocolate. Alternative three, instead of buying a chocolate bar, I will put the money I would have spent towards my next holiday. At 50p a bar I would save over £150 in a year. Now that would cheer me up.)

Question Seven; Ask yourself would any of the three new alternatives be as effective as the original behaviour?

(Example: All three alternatives sound attractive, but I think number one would give me all of the feel good factor I need without the excess calories. In fact knowing that this one thing could help me lose three stone in a year makes me feel even better!*)

* Authors Note. If none of the alternatives are as effective go back to question six. Think carefully and find three different alternatives.

Having carefully reviewed the behaviour that causes you to be overweight, you now know exactly why you behave in this way. More importantly, you now know how to change this behaviour to still get the same benefits, but without the negative side effect of putting on weight.

At this point you are ready for part two and visualise

the difference this new behaviour could make to your life.

Visualise a specific situation where you would have used the old behaviour. Take time to make this image as vivid and realistic as possible. Now switch the old behaviour for your preferred new alternative. Visualise this new situation, and experience how good it makes you feel.

Repeat this visualisation for the other two alternatives.

Now, project yourself a year into the future, visusalise the effect has your new alternative had on your weight.

How much lighter are you?

How does this make you feel?

Visualise yourself in five years time, what difference has your new alternative made to your life?

You would be slimmer, healthier, but is there anything else?

More confidence, increased circle of friends, what difference has it made to your lifestyle?

Having seen the difference your new behaviour could make to your life, you should now do just one more thing. Resolve to take action and make your vision become a reality.

Write down what you are going to do.

CAN YOU SEE THE BLACK AND WHITE TRIANGLES?

*Yes, you see them quite clearly, but they are not really there.
Their shape is only defined by the shape of the other objects,
yet you take this imformation and make sense of it. Your
mind is visualising the shapes.*

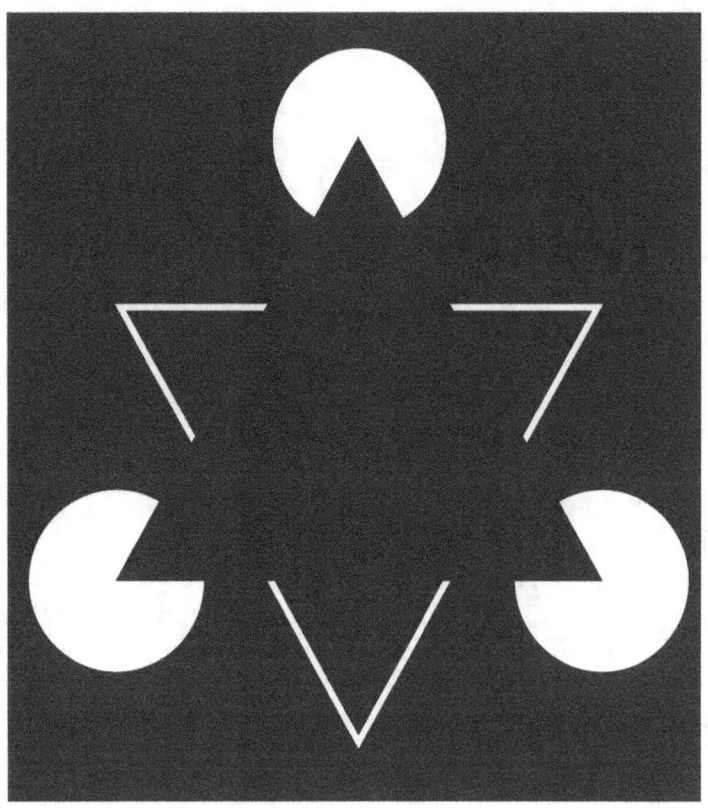

CAN YOU SEE THE BLACK AND WHITE TRIANGLES?

Yes, you see them quite clearly, but they are not really there.
Their shape is only defined by the shape of the other objects,
yet you take this imformation and make sense of it. Your
mind is visualising the shapes.

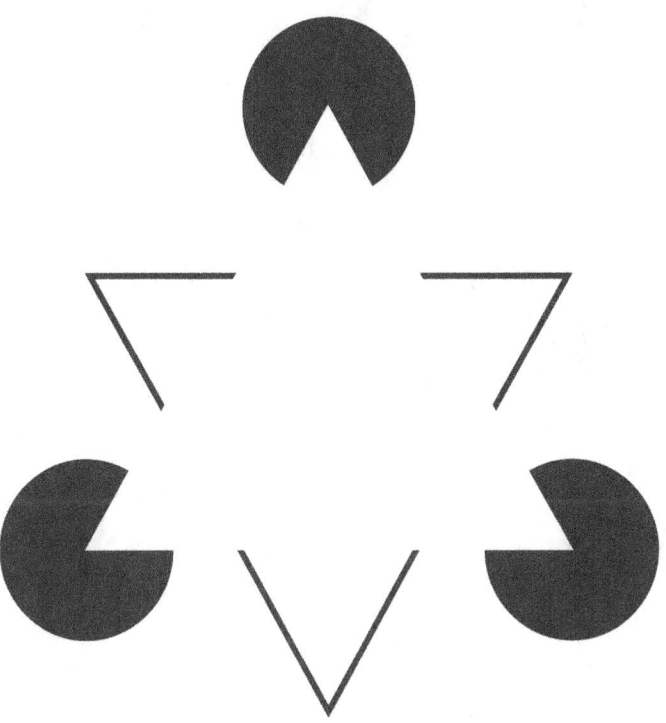

Write it down in the form shown below:

I will
(new alternative one)
instead of
(old behaviour)

I will
(new alternative two)
instead of
(old behaviour)

I will
(new alternative three)
instead of
(old behaviour)

These new alternatives will make
(describe difference)
over a twelve month period.

In five years my life will be
(describe difference).

I resolve to change
(insert old behaviour)
pattern with
(preferred new alternative)
right now.

Diet Shift

The development of the right mental attitude is an essential key to sustainable weight loss. But, in order to live a long and healthy life, reducing your weight is not the only skill you need to master. The foods you eat will not only affect your weight but also your long term health.

C. Norman Shealy MD. PhD, author of The Self-Healing Workbook wrote "*A majority of illnesses have some genetic predilection. Virtually all illnesses, however, are much more strongly influenced by smoking, alcohol, obesity, poor nutrition and inadequate physical exercise than they are by genetics.*"

In recent years the focus on a 'healthy' diet that will keep you free of major illness and will extend your life has been the subject of thousands of reports, scientific studies and books, many of which appear at first sight to be contradictory.

Having studied a great deal of the literature published, I have established that there are common themes on which there is broad agreement. It is these themes that form the basis of this lesson in the programme. If you practice some of these ideas and strategies they will form the foundation for a long, healthy and energetic life. The information provided will give you enough knowledge to help you make your own informed choices on diet and its effect.

Lesson seven the 'Diet Shift' concentrates on two key areas, cholesterol and diet type. These areas are important because you can lose weight and look good outwardly, but still be unhealthy inside.

I have experienced exactly this scenario. About six months after reaching my ideal weight, I happened to have a blood test in which my cholesterol level was checked. The result shocked and scared me. The blood cholesterol level was measured at 221mg or 5.7mmol/l.

Blood cholesterol can be measured in two ways; in millimoles per litre (mmol/l) or in milligrams per decilitre (mg/dl). Millimoles per litre is the standard measurement in the UK. Below is a conversion chart for both measurements.

mg/dl	mmol/l	mg/dl	mmol/l
180	4.66	250	6.47
190	4.91	260	6.72
200	5.17	270	6.98
210	5.43	280	7.24
220	5.69	290	7.50
230	5.95	300	7.76

A measurement of 221mg/dl indicated that my arteries were slowly being blocked by the excess cholesterol. To check this finding I also had an ultrasound scan on the artery in my neck. I could see on the screen in black and white the plaques (cholesterol deposits) that had already built up on the artery wall.

This information gave me a choice, either reduce my cholesterol level or have a high possibility of a heart attack or stroke in my late fifties. My decision was simple and immediate, I changed to a low cholesterol diet. This simply meant avoiding certain types of foods (detailed later) in order to reduce my cholesterol intake.

Three months later, having broadly followed a low cholesterol diet (detailed later) I was re-tested. My blood cholesterol level was down to 170mg or 4.3mmol/l. In just three months I had reduced my possibility of a high cholesterol related illness by 104%.

I was lucky, but many are not, simply because they are not aware of the long term dangers inherent in their existing diet. High cholesterol related illness causes over 40% of all deaths in the U.K. Every year strokes and heart disease kill more people than cancer, yet a small change in diet could dramatically reduce that level. One study that involved over half a million people revealed that a reduction of 21mg or 0.6mmol/l in total cholesterol levels can result in a decrease in the risk of coronary heart disease by as much as 50%.

As a rule of thumb every 1mg reduction in your cholesterol level reduces your chances of suffering from a cholesterol related illness by 2%. So, before we examine low-fat and low cholesterol diets, let us look at cholesterol in more detail.

CHOLESTEROL

Many people think that cholesterol and fat are one and the same thing. They are not. Each has a different effect on the body.

Cholesterol is a waxy, white, fatlike substance, classified as a lipid. It is found in all animal tissues, and is present in all foods produced from animal sources (e.g., eggs, poultry, fish, shellfish and dairy products). Plant based or derived foods do not contain cholesterol.

Cholesterol is needed by the body to produce vitamin D, estrogen and testosterone. Unlike fat you cannot burn it off with exercise. If you have an excess of cholesterol in your blood it will cause your arteries to close. These closures occur when bumps or plaques, grow inside the artery walls. These plaques are simply a build up of cholesterol and will continue to grow, fed by the cholesterol rich blood until eventually the artery is narrowed or blocked. The blood supply is then dramatically reduced or, in extreme cases stopped completely. If you are building up cholesterol in your bloodstream you have a potentially terminal problem.

The only way to reduce your cholesterol level is to consume less. It is possible to look and feel fit and still have a dangerously high cholesterol level.

There are some other very good reasons to reduce your cholesterol levels. High levels of cholesterol in the blood can lead to heart attack, stroke, senility, prostate cancer, cataracts, kidney failure and, in men, impotency.

There are two different types of cholesterol, the good HDL and the bad LDL.

High-density lipoprotein (HDL) is called good because it carries away harmful fatty deposits from cells and other tissues to the liver for excretion from the body. This action helps to prevent the build-up of cholesterol in the walls of your arteries.

Low-density lipoprotein (LDL) accounts for the majority of cholesterol in the blood. It carries cholesterol to the tissues of the body including the arteries. LDL the main source of build-up and blockage in the arteries.

The difference was summed up in a Family Heart Association newsletter: "The HDL are Highly Desirable and the LDL are Less Desirable."

There is also Very low density lipoprotein (VLDL) which are fats that are made in the liver or come from fat in the foods that we eat. They are also known as Triglycerides. Although it is an important source of energy, in excess it can lead to the blood cells clumping to form clots.

WHAT IS A SAFE LEVEL OF CHOLESTEROL?

The American Heart Association recommends that you limit your intake to 300mg/dl per day. The National Cholesterol Education Program recommends no more than 200mg/dl. The Delgado Medical Clinic in California writes

"In populations where artery closure and heart disease are unknown, adults do not have cholesterol levels above 160mg/dl. When we study populations with adult cholesterol levels of 180 to 200, probably 20% have serious artery closure. Populations with levels around 200 to 240 have 100% artery closure. In our country (USA) the average cholesterol level is about 235 to 240."

In England it is estimated that only 30% of the population have a cholesterol level below 200mg/dl or 5.2mmol/l. England is in the world-wide top ten league table for mortality rates from coronary disease. Coincidence? I doubt it.

My first blood test reported a cholesterol count of 221mg/dl or 5.7mmol/l. This would place me in a moderate risk group and therefore not a major cause for concern. Yet an ultrasound of my major arteries revealed evidence of plaque scarring. Based on my experience I recommend a cholesterol level below 170mg or 4.3mmol/l. This means a daily cholesterol intake of less than 120mg per day. (120mg of cholesterol equates to about 4oz of chicken).

I keep my intake of cholesterol low and to do this I choose to avoid certain foods. By avoid I mean that I only eat them occasionally, although it is true that some are consumed more occasionally that others!

The foods that I tend to avoid include;

Poultry/Game   Fried chicken, chicken wings, duck, grouse, egg yolk.

Meat and meat products	Bacon, sausage, liver, pies
Dairy Products	Milk, cream, yoghurt, hard cheeses and butter.
Fish/Seafood	Tuna, salmon, mackerel shrimp.
Others	Chips, cakes, coconut, fried vegetables, chocolate and salad dressings.

At first glance many might consider that avoiding these foods is a little restrictive, so I have outlined two other types of eating plans that will improve your overall levels of health.

All three will make you feel better and help you to eat healthily. I would suggest you look at the three options and consider adapting your existing eating habits to incorporate some aspects of the diets. Have some fun, experiment with them for a period of time see if they make you feel better. I use different elements of all three, which suits my lifestyle and works very effectively.

FAT, FATTER, FATTEST

The are three types of fat that you need to be aware of, Monounsaturated, Polyunsaturated and Saturated fats.

Monounsaturated Fats are usually liquid at room temperature and are found primarily in vegetable products. Current research indicates that monounsaturates have a favourable effect on blood cholesterol levels when consumed in moderation. Examples of foods high in monounsaturated fat are olive oil and peanut oil.

Polyunsaturated Fats are found primarily in vegetable products and are usually liquid at room temperature. When eaten in moderation, polyunsaturated fats have a cholesterol-lowering effect. Examples of foods high in polyunsaturated fat are safflower, sunflower, corn, soybean, cottonseed and margarines made from liquid vegetable oils.

Saturated Fats are usually solid at room temperature. Although they are most commonly found in animal products, saturated fats also occur naturally in such vegetable products as chocolate and coconut. They also occur in vegetable products that have been converted from polyunsaturated fat to a saturated fat through hydrogenation. Examples of foods high in saturated fat are prime cuts of beef, lamb, pork, veal, luncheon meats, poultry skin, lard, butter, whole milk, cream ice cream, cream sauces, cheeses made from whole milk, chocolate, coconut and palm oil. Saturated fat boosts your blood cholesterol level more than anything else in your diet.

LOW FAT DIETS

Fat is generally held responsible for the epidemic proportions of breast, colon and prostate cancer in the major Western countries. When you are overweight, excess fat is found in your blood stream. This excess fat makes the red blood cells clump together and reduces their ability to transport oxygen around the body.

Double Nobel Prize winner Dr Otto Warburg found a link between low oxygen levels in the blood and cancer. He discovered that cells that are deprived of oxygen are more likely to mutate into cancer cells.

The higher the oxygen levels of the blood, the better the chance of avoiding cancer. The oxygen levels in the blood can be increased by deep breathing, exercise and a low fat diet. Studies have shown that a group of marathon runners developed cancer at a rate of 80% less that the general population. The incidence of breast, colon, prostate and other cancers is also decreased in cultures that eat a low fat, high fibre diet.

The most important 'food' for the body is oxygen. Deprive the body of oxygen and it will not survive longer than five to six minutes. To fully oxygenate your body I suggest that you take ten deep breaths at least three times a day.

Try this healthy breathing exercise right now.

1. Take a deep breath for 4 seconds. (Breathe through the nose into the lower abdomen not the chest).

2. Hold it for 4 seconds.

3. Exhale through the mouth for 8 seconds.

4. Repeat 8 times.

How did that feel? You are probably light-headed with all that life giving oxygen rushing around your bloodstream. Repeat this power breathing exercise three times a day and you will soon notice the difference it will make to your overall health and vitality.

So, how low is a low fat diet? The University of California undertook a study of the effects of low-fat diets and concluded "The researchers defined a low fat diet as less that 30% of calories from fat." and added *"Diets consisting of less than 30% of calories from fat have long term health benefits by helping to prevent chronic diseases and establishing healthful eating habits."*

The figure of 30% or less of calories from fat, with less than 10% from saturated fat, has been universally accepted as the definition of a low fat diet.

Start to read the labels on the foods you buy at the supermarket, look for the fat content, then think carefully before buying anything with a 15% fat content or above. I use the figure of 15% for two reasons: Firstly, there are many hidden fats in our diet which have to be accounted for, and more importantly 15% gives a margin of error for those occasional binges.

There are many guidelines on low fat available should you wish to research the area in more detail. If not, here are some simple tips that will help:

Make fish, turkey and chicken your main source of non-vegetable protein. Eat more complex carbohydrates (fruits), coarse-grained breads, whole wheat, bran cereals and raw or lightly steamed vegetables.

Substitute butter on bread for a low fat spread. Consider alternatives to frying or using oil, use a Wok or skillet with a non stick cooking spray.

On the following pages are two useful charts. The first is a list of foods, with a recommended usage based on a low fat diet. The second is a similar chart specifically for cheese. I'm sure you will find them useful.

FOOD COMBINING OR THE HAY SYSTEM DIET

The Food Combining or Hay System was devised by the American Doctor William Howard Hay in the 1920's. At 40 years of age he was severely overweight and in failing health, he was suffering from a serious kidney condition, high blood pressure and an enlarged heart. He was deemed as untreatable by the medical services of the day. Spurred on by a desire to live beyond his early 40's he created a new, uncomplicated method of eating, which he believed allowed the body's natural healing powers to work to their maximum effect. He felt that disease resulted from the accumulation of toxins in the body. The Hay System was devised to restore a natural balance to the body. Using this system Dr Hay reduced his weight by 50lbs, eradicated his heart and kidney problems and reduced his blood pressure to normal. He also lived to a respectable old age.

The Hay system works on the basis that ill health is a product of the accumulation of toxins in the body, which in turn, is caused by four main factors:

	EAT REGULARLY	EAT IN MODERATION OR OCCASIONALLY	EAT IN MODERATION OR AS A TREAT	AVOID THESE FOODS
CEREAL	Wholemeal flour, Oatmeal, Wholemeal bread, Whole grain cereal, Porridge, Oats, Crispbreads, Brown Rice, Wholemeal Pasta, Cornmeal, Sugar-free muesli, Rice cakes.	White bread, White flour, White rice/pasta, Water biscuits, Wholemeal scones, Oat scones, Teacakes, Pancake.	Sugar-coated cereals, Plain semi-sweet biscuits, Ordinary muesli.	Sweet biscuits, Cream-filled biscuits, Cream Crackers, Cheese biscuits, Croissants.
FRUIT AND VEGETABLES	All fresh fruit, Dried or frozen fruit, Unsweetened tinned fruit, vegetables, Baked potatoes, Tofu.	Olives, Oven Chips (cooked in sunflower oil), Avocado.	Fruit in syrup, Crystallized fruit, Chips & roast potatoes (cooked in suitable oil).	Deep fat fried chips, Roast potatoes, Crisps & savoury snacks.
NUTS	Chestnuts, Walnuts, Pinenuts.	Pistachio, Pecan, Almonds, Sesame seeds, Sunflower seeds.	Peanuts, All nuts not mentioned.	Coconut.
FISH	All fresh or frozen fish.	Fish fried in suitable oil, Grilled fish fingers, Grilled fish cakes.	Prawns, Lobster, Crab, Oysters, molluscs, Winkles, Fish tinned in oil.	Fish roe, Taramasalata, Fried scampi.
MEAT	Chicken (No skin), Turkey (No skin), Veal, Rabbit, Game, Soya meat substitute, Lean red meat.	Lean Beef, Pork, Lamb, Ham, Gammon, Lean minced Beef.	Liver, Kidney, Tripe, Sweetbreads, Grilled Back Bacon, Duck (No skin), Low fat pate.	Sausages, Luncheon meat, Corned Beef, Pate, Salami, Streaky Bacon, Burgers, Goose, Meat Pies, Sausage Rolls, Pasties, Scotch Eggs, Meat Fat, Crackling, Skin.
PREPARED FOODS	Jelly (low sugar), Sorbet, Fat free homemade soups.	Pastry, Puddings, Cakes, Biscuits, Sauces etc. (with fat or oil as below), Low fat ready prepared meals.	Packet soups, Non Dairy ice cream, Custard mix (made with water or skimmed milk).	Pastries, Puddings, cakes and sauces (with whole milk or fat or oil as below), Suet, Cream soups.

	EAT REGULARLY	EAT IN MODERATION OCCASIONALLY	EAT IN MODERATION AS A TREAT	AVOID EATING
EGGS & DAIRY PRODUCTS	Skimmed milk, Soya milk, Cottage cheese, Low fat curd cheese, Low fat yoghurt, Egg white, Low fat fromage frais.	Semi-skimmed milk, Whole eggs (three in total).	Medium fat cheeses (see cheese chart), Half fat cheeses. Sweetened condensed skimmed milk.	Whole milk, Cream, Full fat yoghurt, Full fat cheeses (see cheese chart), Evaporated milk, condensed milk, Imitation cream, More than four whole eggs per week.
FATS	Fat Substitute	Margarine (high in Polyunsaturates or monounsaturates), Corn oil, Sunflower oil, Soya oil, Safflower oil, Grapeseed oil, Olive oil, Peanut oil, Reduced fat and low fat spreads.		All margarines and oils (that are not high in polyunsaturates or monounsaturates), Butter, Lard, Suet, Dripping, Vegetable oil, Spreads (not labled low fat).
SWEETS, JAMS, PRESERVES & SPREADS	Marmite, Bovril, Chutney, Pickles, Sugar free sweeteners, Low sugar jams and marmalade.	Fish & Meat paste, Peanut butter, Jam, Marmalade, Honey, Low fat soft cheese, Low fat spreads.	Boiled sweets, fruit pastiles & jellies.	Chocolate spreads, Chocolate, toffees, fudge, butterscotch, Carob chocolate, Coconut bars
DRINKS	Fresh Tea, Coffee (in limited amounts), mineral water, fruit juice (unsweetened).	Alcohol	Sweetened drinks, squashes, fruit juice, Malted milk, Hot chocolate drinks (with skimmed milk).	Whole milk drinks, Cream based liqueurs. Coffee whitener.
SAUCES AND DRESSINGS	Herbs, spices, Tabasco, Worcestershire sauce, Soy sauce, Lemon juice, Garlic, Pepper.	Homemade salad dressings & mayonnaise (with oils from above)	Low fat or low calorie mayonnaises & dressings. Parmesan cheese.	Ordinary cream dressings & mayonnaises.

Until you have reached a desired weight, foods high in sugar should be avoided and intake of suitable fats and oils strictly limited. EAT REGULARLY means that you can choose from this group daily (limiting meat and fish to 4-5 ounces per day). EAT IN MODERATION OCCASIONALLY means moderate amounts 2-3 times per week. A TREAT is a small amount once a week.

1. Eating too many refines foods, starches and acid-forming proteins.

2. Poor elimination of toxins and wastes.
3. Not eating enough alkaline-forming vegetables and fruits.

4. The mixing of incompatible foods, especially starches and proteins.

Foods are then classified into three types according to their chemical requirements for digestion. The three food types are;

Alkali-forming foods. These are defined as alkali-forming because this is their final state after digestion. Fruit and vegetables fall into this category, even 'acid' tasting fruits such as lemons produce alkaline salts in the body.

Concentrated proteins. Are acid-forming when digested and include meat, game, eggs, cheese and fish.

Concentrated carbohydrates and starch. These are also acid forming and include all foods that contain flour, grains and bread. Also classified in this category are sugars, or foods containing sugar, except naturally occurring sugars as found in fruit.

The essential message of the Hay System is to avoid combining foods that need conflicting chemicals to digest them. This conflict leads to inefficient or partial digestion, or put more technically:

"Each kind of food provokes a specific, definite type of gastric and intestinal secretion. Because the presence of the three concentrated foods calls for antagonistic chemical processes at the same time, it is a physical and chemical impossibility for the digestive glands to function properly, as they are subject to definite physiological laws." N. Philip Norman, M.D, Lecturer in Gastroenterology, New York Medical School and Hospital.

Another key message of the Hay System is that the body contains alkaline and acid mineral salts in the proportion of four to one. To maintain a natural balance we should eat foods that maintain this balance. If an imbalance of these foods are consumed, it upsets the mineral balance of the body which contributes to ill-health.

To follow the Hay System, there are five rules that you need to remember;

Rule One. Don't mix foods that fight ie; starches and sugars do not mix with proteins and acid fruits. Do not eat them at the same time. Following this rule will help you to digest food in the most efficient way. Digestion is the largest energy drain on the human body, so making this process as efficient as possible has the side-effect of raising your energy levels. It will also increase your general level of health.

Rule Two. Vegetables, fruit and salads should form the major part of your diet. The body is composed of 70% water; most vegetables, fruits and salads are composed of 70% water. Eating these foods on a regular basis will keep the body fluids in balance.

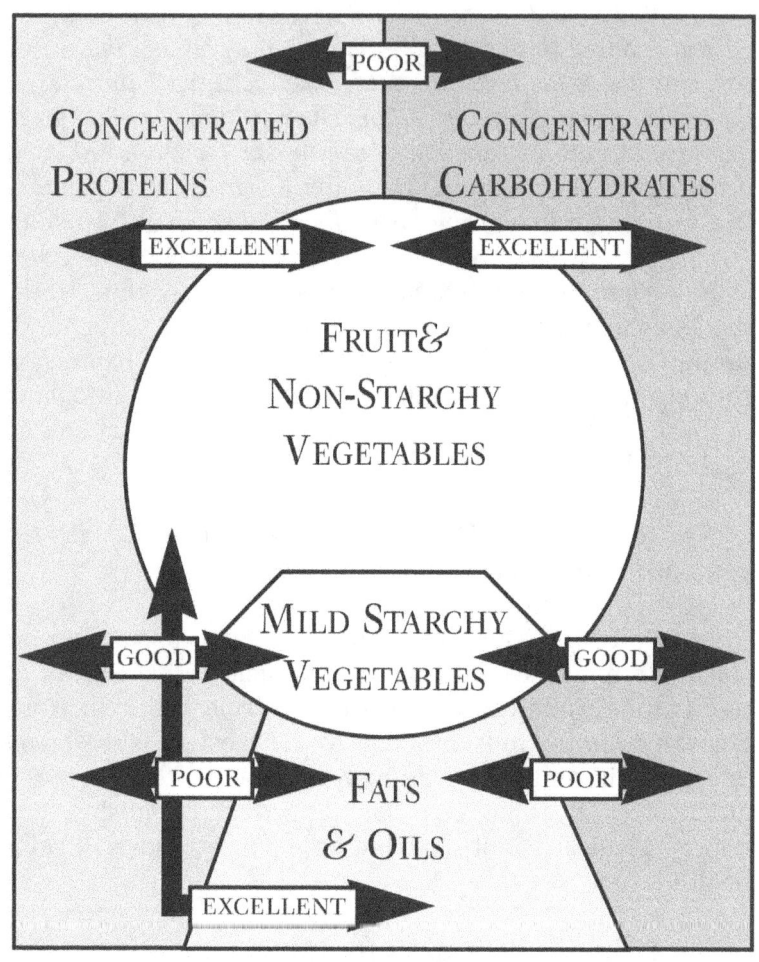

Rule Three. Cut down on proteins, starches and fats which should only constitute 20% of your diet.

Rule Four. Refined and processed foods should be cut out of your diet. These should be replaced by whole grains and unprocessed starches. Avoid white flour and sugar, processed fats, margarine, and sweetened foods and drinks.

Rule Five. Four hours should pass between meals of starches/sugars and proteins/acid fruits.

Many people who use the Hay System report being less tired and having more energy because of the increased efficiency of the digestive process. They also report that they don't feel bloated or heavy stomached after a meal, and that they sleep better at night. Again this is probably because the digestive process is not working overtime trying to digest conflicting foods.

Alongside is a chart that summarises the dos and don'ts of the Hay System.

VERY LOW FAT, LOW CHOLESTEROL

A very Low Fat diet is one where you limit your intake of fat to under 15% of your calorie intake per day. This can be done by eating foods with a fat content of less than 10%. To achieve this you would also need complex carbohydrates to make up 70% of your normal daily intake.

A low cholesterol diet is one in which you restrict your cholesterol intake to less than 100mg per day. The easiest way to achieve this is to avoid eating any animal, animal by-products and dairy products. The Delgado Clinic in California, who are acknowledged world leaders in methods of cholesterol reduction suggest "To rapidly reduce your cholesterol level, prepare your meals without any type of meat as often as possible."

This advice is much easier to follow that many people think. There are many excellent vegetarian variations of popular meat dishes available, and increasingly since the concerns over public consumption of meat, especially beef, the many superb soya and quorn based meat substitutes have become very popular. If you have not already tried them I urge you to do so.

There are other foods which are high in cholesterol which are listed, with their cholesterol content; Egg yolks contain 1,500mg per 100grammes, Whole eggs 500mg, Liver 300mg, Butter 250mg, Shrimp 160mg, Crab 100mg, Cheese 100mg, Mackerel 95mg, Veal 90mg, Turkey 82 mg, Lobster 82mg, Beef 68mg, Pork 68mg, Lamb 68mg, Salmon 68mg, Tuna 63mg, Chicken 60mg, Whole Milk 11mg, Skimmed Milk 3mg. These foods should be eaten occasionally or avoided.

The good news is that all Grains, Fruits, Vegetables, Pulses, Nuts and seeds contain no cholesterol so you can enjoy them on a regular basis.

LOOKING GOOD

Men tend to look their best with a body fat level of between 15 and 18%, for women the figure is slightly higher at between 18 and 22%. It seems perfectly logical to me that to reach this figure our intake of fat should not exceed those higher limits. The body can only release more fat from the cells than it stores if there is less fat in your diet.

Exercise will make a difference, if you workout three times a week and for at least thirty minutes this will keep your metabolic rate up and help to burn of excess calories.

If you do decide to exercise on a regular basis, totally ignore the "No pain, No gain" principle. It is not necessary to over exert yourself to gain the full benefits of regular exercise. In fact pushing yourself too hard is counter productive because your body will burn its sugar reserves instead of its stored fat.

As a rule of thumb when exercising your heartrate should not exceed 180 beats per minute minus your age. For example for a forty year old the ideal heartrate while exercising is 140 beats per minute (180-40 = 140). One way to tell if you are exceeding your comfort zone is by listening to your breathing, if you are gasping for breath you are working too hard. Ease off, and enjoy

If you choose to reduce your fat intake in your diet to under 15% you will see a dramatic reduction of your weight in the medium to long term.

In the short term you could temporarily see a slight weight increase. This is because while you lose body fat you will gain water. This is because the reduction of fat in the diet allows more glycogen into your muscles. Glycogen absorbs three grams of additional water for each additional gram of glycogen. This re-hydration of the body has a useful side effect as it will help improve your general muscle and body tone. To aid this process it is recommended that you drink at least 6 to 8 glasses of water per day. This re-hydration process has a number of positive benefits; it will make you feel better, it will improve the liver and kidney functions, it helps to suppress your appetite and help you to lose weight.

LIVE LONG AND PROSPER

Diet Shift has only one goal which is to give you some diet choices which will enable you to live a longer, happier healthier life. In a study that examined over 100 million people in 25 countries who follow a diet which is high in fibre and complex carbohydrates and low in fat and cholesterol, almost no killer diseases such as heart disease were found. Incidents of cancer were below expected averages and life expectancy past the age of 40 was higher.

If the sentiment of the No Diet-Diet is think yourself slimmer, the sentiment of Diet Shift is eat yourself fitter. I urge you to consider some simple changes that you could make to your diet right now and suggest that you to take action. Make a small change right now, it could be the beginning of a new leaner, healthier you.

When temptation strikes

There will come a time when, despite all of the positive strategies you have developed, you will sooner or later have an overwhelming desire to eat something that will just pile on the pounds. Don't worry, this is a perfectly natural reaction. Just because you have traded an old set of behaviours for a new improved set does not mean that they have disappeared. The old behaviours will surface from time to time, in moments of stress or when your achievements overtake your self image.

Agatha McFarlane, having successfully lost two stone in three months, recalls the pressure from her peer group "Most of my friends and colleagues are happy for me and compliment me. The flip side is that others, while being curious as to how I have accomplished this, cannot help saying something discouraging. One needs a strong belief in oneself, otherwise it would be very easy to get deflated and return to the past."

Remember the tale of Michael Hebranko, who lost over 57 stone and despite reaching his goal put most of it back on in less than eighteen months. This happened because Micheal failed to properly address the psychological aspects of weight loss. His self image was still that of an overweight man trapped in a thin body. He then simply succumb to the urges to eat in a subconscious effort to make his body conform to his self image. This uses exactly the same strategies and principles of this programme except in reverse.

Apart from the enormous amount of weight he lost, he was an unusual case in as much that he reached his goal before he started to get urges to binge. This happens in an estimated 9% of cases. Usually most people break their diets long before reaching their goal weight.

If you get the urge to binge that's great! Have fun. Enjoy it. Don't feel guilty. In my view you should deny yourself nothing, but what you should do is moderate and consciously control these eating tendencies.

The best long term diet strikes the right balance between healthy eating and the occasional irrational indulgence. The problem with the diet of most overweight people is that they have just tipped the scales too far the wrong way.

I have developed an eight point strategy that I use when I'm being, or intend to be, over indulgent. The strategy can be used to plan an indulgence or as a fall back position for an unplanned binge.

BINGEING STRATEGY

1. Realise it's happening. This is most important, if you do not know when you are being over indulgent, it is hard to take positive steps to control the situation.

2. Understand exactly why it's happening. Rationalise the circumstances behind the desire to eat the wrong foods. It could be the circumstances, for example a social gathering. It could be because you are feeling low. Whatever the reason if you should understand the motivation behind the behaviour, then it is easier to modify. Use affirmations, they are very good for changing behaviour.

3. Accept the situation and the consequences. OK you have pigged out. You have over indulged yourself, don't regret this after the event. All you have done is traded the indulgence for a minor time delay in reaching the ideal you. Accept the trade.

4. Set a specific time limit. You need to quantify when your indulgence will end. This is important, a failure to do this can signal the return of previous eating behaviours on a more permanent basis.

5. Enjoy it while it lasts. Savour your indulgence, make the most of it, but remember you are only able to enjoy it and move towards your ideal weight because of the way you eat usually.

6. Stop at the pre-determined point. Don't be tempted to continue after your pre-determined finish point. Put the indulgence to one side, it will always be there and you can come back to it another time.

7. Resolve to rectify the effect. Return to eating in a way that causes you to move towards your goal. I have a rule of thumb that seems to work very well, I eat sensibly for at least 90% of the time and have small indulgence 10% of the time. Or, to put itanother way reserve one or two meals a week for your indulgences.

8. Take positive action. Monitor your progress and reduce or increase your indulgence time dependant on the results you are getting. Remember that not losing weight is your body's way of telling you to reduce them.

Most people tend to binge if they are hungry. If we eat when we are hungry, we tend to overeat, and overeat things that are not good for us. There is a simple solution to this, don't let yourself get hungry. Eat on a regular basis. Yes, I am suggesting that your eat between meals and there is a very good reason why you should.

Most complex carbohydrates take about one hour to be digested, the sugars distributed via the bloodstream and converted to energy by the muscles. So if you eat fruit or vegetables it is logical and advisable to eat every hour. Grains and pulses take around two hours to go through this process. If you fast for much longer than two hours your blood sugar levels become depleted and you start to feel tired, irritable and hungry.

This is when you become prone to overeating. There is a simple technique that you can use to 'listen' to your body and help you to eat before you get to this point. With a little practice, it is easy to tell how hungry you are. Try this technique right now, to tell when you next need to eat.

THE FUEL TANK TECHNIQUE

Imagine that your stomach is like the fuel tank of a car. Imagine that it has a fuel gauge, which reads either full, three quarters full, half full, a quarter full or empty.

Full means that your stomach is so full that it is bloated and uncomfortable. Three quarters full gives you a satisfied and comfortable feeling. Half full gives you no sensation of being full or hungry. Quarter full is when you feel empty inside and feel the initial need for food and empty is when you are very hungry and feel a desperate need to eat.

To find out where your fuel gauge is right now, just place your hand over your stomach. Take three deep breaths to relax and imagine that you can see the fuel gauge in front of you. Where is your needle pointing?

Now that you know how to read the gauge, here are some tips on how to use it. You should avoid eating so much that you are full (this is how 80% of people put on weight in the first place). You should aim to fill your tank to three quarters full. You should always eat something when the tank is a quarter full and never let it run to empty.

If you follow this simple set of guidelines, you'll be amazed how quickly you will lose weight. This is a good technique to use before you eat, as you will quickly discover that in seven out of ten instances you don't really need to eat at all. Most of the eating we do is driven by habit or social conditioning, and rarely has anything to do with our needs. This technique, if used on a regular basis, will show you exactly how often you eat unnecessarily.

Just do it!

THE IMPORTANCE OF FAILURE

Most people fear failure, they see it as something to be avoided, something to be ashamed of. This attitude comes from not fully understanding the important part that failure plays in success.

There is a story about Thomas Eddison that highlights the importance of understanding the nature of failure. Thomas Eddison was the inventor of the electric light. He was also the most successful inventor of his time, with over 500 patents registered. He also had the largest number of failed scientific experiments to his credit.

While Thomas Eddison was trying to create the carbon impregnated filament, (the basis for electric light), a young reporter came to see him. It is worth remembering at this point in time the world was lit by kerosene lamps. The young reporter asked Eddison why he persisted with his futile experiments, as he'd already had over 5,000 failures. Eddison is reported to have replied "You don't understand the way the world works. I have not failed 5,000 times. I have successfully identified 5,000 ways which will not work.

That puts me exactly 5,000 ways closer to the one that does." Eventually, some 4,000 experiments later, Eddison found the way that worked and the electric light was born.

The Eddison example is by no means unusual. There are many examples of business people who experience their greatest successes immediately after their worst failures.

Failure is a pre-requisite to success. It's not how far you fall, it's how high you bounce that counts. When you understand the nature of failure, you actually welcome it because failure always contains a valuable lesson that will take you that much closer to success next time around.

Right at the beginning of this programme I said *"If you have tried and failed to lose weight in the past, that past failure is actually an advantage! Your previous attempts to lose weight have not been wasted. You will have learnt from the experience. You will have gained a valuable insight into how not to approach the subject of weight loss - and you are less likely to make the same mistakes again. In one of the few comprehensive studies conducted on weight loss, it was found that people who had been unsuccessful in losing weight in the past were 20% more likely succeed in the future."*

THE PAST DOES NOT EQUAL THE FUTURE

Just because your efforts to lose weight have not had the desired effect previously does not mean that it will always be that way. All that you need to do is re-evaluate your approach and try something a little different. The important thing is that you try something else. If you take no positive action, you will see no positive result.

If you are serious about losing weight, commit now to taking a positive action. Choose one or more of the six actions below and just do it!

1. Resolve to lose one ounce a day.

Change just one thing in your existing diet that will help you lose on ounce a day. And stick to it for at least 30 days.

2. Go on a 21 day positive affirmation diet.

Pick your favourite affirmations from "Think yourself slimmer', or better still make up some of your own. Use them on a daily basis, especially when you feel temptation may strike.

3. Accept responsibility for your actions.

You present weight accurately reflects the decisions you have taken previously about your eating habits. From now on there are no more excuses.

4. Travel the weight escalator.

Visualise yourself as slimmer, imagine the positive effect this will have on your life. Think about this potential future on a regular basis and use these feelings to built up your motivation to make that future a reality.

5. Listen to the 'tip and affirmations' audio.

There are times when reading is difficult, so consider listening to the audio when you are in the car, or in the evening when you are relaxed.

6. Before you next eat, use the fuel tank technique.

This will help you to determine if you really need to eat or not.

HIT A WINNER

To make this programme work you must take action. If you study this programme, find it interesting and then just put it on a shelf to gather dust, the chances are that you will still be at your existing weight in a year from now. To change you must take action.

Taking action has been likened to the game of rounders. Think of it as an analagy for your desire to lose weight. In rounders, you have three strikes at the ball before you are out.

We all play the rounders game of life, but if you are determined and take action you can change the rules and the result in your favour. You can become the umpire as well as the batsman. As umpire you can change the rules to suit yourself.

You can decide how long to stand in the batting square. You can take a swing at as many deliveries as you like and as the umpire only you can decide when to call yourself out.

By focussing on being determined and taking action you can swing at the deliveries all day and by the law of averages you will eventually hit the ball out of the park. If you resolve to take action and stick with it you will suceed where 98% of people fail. You will achieve your ideal weight.

Use the techniques in this programme and, like many people who have used its techniques and strategies before you, you will hit a home run and lose weight. There is no great secret. It is simply a question of determination, confidence and application.

I know this to be true. The people who have used the techniques described in this programme know it to be true.

In your heart you know it too, you can achieve anything when you have set your mind to it. You are unique. You are special. You can be, do or achieve whatever you believe with conviction. You can be slim and stay slim for the rest of your life. Mentally I suspect that you are already losing weight.

Now, all that you have to do is to pick up the bat and keep swinging until you hit that ball out of the park.

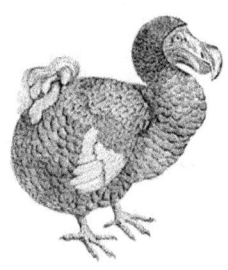